Improve Eyesight

How to Naturally Improve Your Vision Through Simple Eye Exercises

(Improve Your Vision Naturally Without Glasses, Lenses or Surgery)

Terry Young

Published By **Chris David**

Terry Young

Improve Eyesight: How to Naturally Improve Your Vision Through Simple Eye Exercises (Improve Your Vision Naturally Without Glasses, Lenses or Surgery)

ISBN   978-1-998769-80-3

Legal & Disclaimer

Table Of Contents

Chapter 1: What Is Natural Vision Improvement (Nvi)?

Can Your Optometrist Or Eye Doctor Be Trusted With The Entirety Of Your Eye Health?

When you visit your optometrist, you will commonly take delivery of 3 alternatives: eyewear, medication or surgical operation. There is however a completely specialized department of optometry that uses herbal imaginative and prescient improvement methods. It is a traditional shape of medical doctor-led remedy referred to as 'imaginative and prescient therapy'. Most optometrists and eye medical doctors aren't knowledgeable in imaginative and prescient therapy. Despite all the medical proof, many even agree with that imaginative and prescient therapy doesn't work, however this is most effective due to the fact they're uninformed about it.

Eye doctors are exceptional in relation to diagnosing eye sickness and performing surgical operation on the eyes. They are but, generally under-informed with reference to visual processing, accommodation, convergence and vision remedy. Many will admit to this. Dr David Guyton, eye muscle physician and researcher, wrote in the clinical magazine, Transactions of the American Ophthalmological Society: "We (ophthalmologists) have in all likelihood abdicated the examine of lodging and convergence to the optometric profession. A perusal of the literature will screen that maximum of the advances in this location are being made in the optometric establishments through vision scientists who use definitions and terms with which we are not even familiar."

Vision remedy is a completely specialized field of traditional optometry that most optometrists and eye docs recognise little or no approximately.

Think approximately it. If most medical doctors/optometrists don't agree with in traditional, scientifically demonstrated, physician-led vision remedy because of a loss of training on their element, even fewer nevertheless could consider in natural imaginative and prescient development techniques that you can practice in your own.

So if your eye physician tells you that the non-surgical approach doesn't work, don't forget that he/she has little know-how on the subject. Doctors who criticize vision therapy and natural imaginative and prescient improvement have not executed their homework. Since maximum eye doctors and optometrists aren't educated in both discipline, there may be no factor in requesting their reviews on herbal vision development.

If you need to study imaginative and prescient remedy, you need to technique an optometrist who specializes in imaginative and prescient therapy. If you want to find out about natural imaginative and prescient improvement, you have to approach a herbal imaginative and prescient development therapist.

Generally speakme, behavioral optometrists who specialise in vision remedy have a few information of herbal vision development and understand that it can work (because the two varieties of therapy have a lot in common). However, even imaginative and prescient therapists are possibly to inform you that herbal imaginative and prescient development doesn't work. Why? The motive here is typically cash.

Let me give an explanation for.

We want to see fitness-care experts as all being obtainable with the sole goal to serve the extra desirable – as in moral, humanitarian people who commit their lives to assisting others with out looking anything in return.

Although I actually have seen this to be the case with a very small handful of medical doctors in society, the full-size majority are extra influenced by means of money, social reputation and electricity than the average patient would ever believe.

In a 1993 survey of eye muscle surgeons, Paul Romano, MD, the editor of Eye Muscle Surgery Quarterly, asked surgeons throughout the globe a query. The surgeons have been requested whether or not they could opt for a surgical or a non-surgical method to the treatment of intermittent exotropia (a sort of strabismus). Where eighty five% of international eye surgeons recommended non-surgical techniques, handiest fifty two% of American surgeons did the equal. Dr Romano suggested there were 3 motives why greater American surgeons preferred surgical operation than non-American surgeons.

1. Insurance groups out of doors the U.S. Do not pay as properly for eye muscle surgical procedure than insurance corporations in the U.S.

2. Surgical remedy is more economically profitable in the U.S. Than non-surgical therapy.

3. Due to the lack of education in non-surgical therapy, surgeons inside the U.S. Are reluctant to well known its advantages in worry of dropping patients.

The optometric enterprise is a multi-billion dollar industry. It is developing extremely rapid as more and more humans are wearing glasses and having laser eye therapy to improve their vision. The complete industry, with all of the corporate fat cats at the pinnacle, want you to maintain shopping for glasses for the relaxation of your life, as your imaginative and prescient keeps to deteriorate, hoping that at the give up of it you may spend many lots of dollars on having laser eye surgery.

Optometry is a multi-billion dollar industry this is developing every yr, as an increasing number of human beings are sporting glasses. NVI is possibly the most important danger the industry has ever faced.

According to the Vision Council of America, about seventy five% of adults wear corrective lenses - that makes for a hell of a big enterprise. But as illustrated inside the examine above, it isn't always just the men at the top that want you to continue sporting glasses, your optometrist wishes this as well.

According to the American Optometric Association, the average optometrist operating in an workplace makes over $96,000 in line with 12 months as of 2008.

Self-employed optometrists common approximately $175,000 according to 12 months. There's absolute confidence that the self-employed optometrist cashes in big time every time a affected person is satisfied to shop for a couple glasses. What you may not recognize but, is that optometrists in a profits process are given economic incentives for making you wear glasses. The greater of their patients who purchase glasses, the extra they receives a commission.

Knowing this, what number of optometrists do you think will inform you that you do not really want glasses? That you may opposite your visible deterioration with a easy set of eye sporting activities? After that you are probable to mention some thing along the strains of 'Wow, I had no idea I ought to try this, tell me how!' The negative optometrist could then be obliged to spend a great short while of his time explaining the character of natural imaginative and prescient improvement to you with NO financial compensation in anyway. If he did this with all of his sufferers, he would quickly be the poorest optometrist on the town.

So I desire you're getting the message right here. No health practitioner/optometrist is ever probably to inform you the reality about herbal vision development. As with most herbal and alternative forms of remedy, you need to do your own research and strive it out for yourself to know whether or not it works or now not. There's no factor in asking a physician who's skilled simplest in conventional scientific/surgical remedy. The handiest reason you should bring up the topic of herbal or opportunity therapy together with your health practitioner is to test whether or not it's miles safe to your specific scenario.

Enter William H Bates

Speaking of skilled docs, the idea of the use of exercising and alternative techniques to help regain clear eyesight turned into first counseled by way of William Horatio Bates. He posited that every one sight issues are due to routine pressure of the eyes and that glasses had been harmful and pointless. And thus the Bates Method – the forerunner of Natural Vision Improvement – turned into conceived in 1920.

Bates' principle become, of direction, now not best. Some of the packages of his theories have been instead risky, like searching immediately on the solar on the way to help loosen up the eyes. Another dangerous principle became the total dismissal of optical glasses – which can be pretty risky if the person doing so has not completely recovered his or her imaginative and prescient simply but. In fact, it is taken into consideration unlawful for people with impaired vision to pressure on the road if they do no longer wear their prescription glasses.

But this does not mean that Bates became absolutely off the mark.

The theories he proposed touched on herbal, instinctive human reactions to eye pain. For example, why can we rub our eyes when they're angry? Why can we near them while we were studying books or watching TV for prolonged periods of time? Why is it that looking at distant, inexperienced gadgets helps ease the tension in our eyes after prolonged use? Why does a water-cooled towel laid out on our eyes sense so darned proper after a long day on the workplace?

And then there are the cognitive – the notion-related – components of seeing. We can educate ourselves to do a number of tasks that contain the usage of our eyes: noting spelling errors even as proofreading a file, monitoring whoever has the ball when Super Bowl season comes rolling across the nook, recognizing that preferred emblem of chips inside the grocery store aisle and so much more. So why can't we educate ourselves to use our eyes now not only for one unique mission however to 'see' better at whatever we want to?

Bates had thus pointed out each physical and cognitive answers to eye issues, and this is wherein Natural Vision Improvement is available in.

Natural Vision Improvement (or NVI) is a present day edition of the Bates Method, keeping and enhancing the theories which have been located to paintings even as enhancing or getting rid of the ones which have been located to be not as effective as to start with thought to be.

Modern NVI revolves round five foremost ideas: (1) bodily enjoyable the eyes, (2) physically strengthening the eyes, (3) 'getting to know' how to see better, (4) nourishing your eyes and (5) developing better imaginative and prescient-related habits.

1. Physically Relaxing The Eyes

Physical relaxation of the eye is the most effective and maximum direct aspect of Natural Vision Improvement.

This involves doing diverse activities which loosen up the muscle tissue and nerves that control the eye. These parts of the attention are responsible for controlling how we circulate our eyes and how we interpret the optical alerts our eyes acquire. Relaxing the eyes thus offers them time to recover from the constant stress we divulge them to, in addition to priming them for the following step of the NVI plan.

2. Physically Strengthening The Eyes

That next step is the physical strengthening of the attention.

This involves workout the muscle groups that manipulate our eyeballs, in addition to strengthening the neurological pathways wherein indicators from the eye travel to the mind. These sporting activities help enhance notion, tracking and attention – three number one aspects of imaginative and prescient that many people take for granted in their each day lives. Training the muscle tissue and nerves on your eyes can for that reason sharpen your vision, particularly while you discover ways to better 'see' the matters around you rather than just 'looking' at them.

This is wherein mastering how to see better comes in...

three. Learning How To See Better

What we see is colored by what is going on in our head, specifically when we're in an emotionally-charged scenario like a heated argument, a shocking shock or a easy loss of challenge. This is why it's miles critical that we all learn how to see matters for what they may be instead of just searching blindly at what unfolds earlier than us. This is why we discover ways to see better with the aid of figuring out and handling common "seeing" styles that prevent us from seeing our environment.

Then you do, of path, must well nourish your eyes with the proper kinds of meals...

four. Nourishing Your Eyes With Good Nutrition

Your eyes are an imperative part of your body, and you need to devour the right form of food to preserve your eyes sturdy and wholesome.

You'll find more element on imaginative and prescient boosting meals later on this e book, however for now, recognize that you need to devour plenty of colored vegetables, particularly the ones darkish greens.

There are also positive meals that do more to heal and toughen your eyes, and may be pretty beneficial whilst you're schooling your eyes. They are not one-shot miracle treatment options, although. They are easy foodstuffs which can boost up the system and hold your eyes higher controlled in the long-run.

One first-rate instance is the Indian spice turmeric. If you need to improve your vision, you'll go an extended manner with the aid of getting your self a exquisite turmeric complement for protective your eyes and boosting vision inside the lengthy-run. Here's one that is working properly for me and for my clients:

Click here (U.S. Handiest)

And in the end you have the conduct that can promote sharper imaginative and prescient even as minimizing eye harm...

five. Developing Better Vision-Related Habits

There are two sorts of habits: bad behavior and top behavior.

Bad eye behavior positioned more pressure on the eyes than they are able to manage. Straining the muscle groups of the eyes can impair your vision each inside the quick-run and in the lengthy-run.

Good eye habits, alternatively, supply your eyes the relaxation they want even as enhancing your capacity to see better. We intention to cultivate the latter and cast off the previous on this guide.

NVI is a holistic integration of the physical, physiological and mental improvement of the eyes. This places it squarely inside the class of opportunity remedy, which brings us to the subsequent bankruptcy of our guide: how exactly does NVI engage with current optometry?

Seeing is a complex system that includes the eyes, brain, and the eye-brain neuronal connection. All 3 ought to paintings in ideal harmony to provide you with clean imaginative and prescient. Any precise NVI software will subsequently have a multi-faceted method that addresses all three of these components of visual processing

THE ROLE OF NVI IN MAINSTREAM OPTOMETRY

As noted within the previous bankruptcy, Natural Vision Improvement is an opportunity shape of eye therapy. Its equivalent in mainstream medicine is optometry.

Optometrists (aka ophthalmic opticians) awareness on diagnosing eye situations, undertaking eye surgery, prescribing optical aids, and prescribing drugs. In brief, they are the contemporary, conventional specialists in something that worries imaginative and prescient and the eyes. Optometrists are the parents excellent capable of coping with critical eye situations, and are valuable with regards to the safety of your eyes.

But there are quite a few problems with mainstream optometry – in particular for the average Joe and Jane together with his or her personal set of unique occasions.

The first and most obvious trouble right here is the money concerned.

Optometrists address the answer via prescribing the fastest and maximum truthful solutions to the situation. The common pair of glasses best takes an hour or so to fabricate, whilst a prescription shape may be speedy filled and handed out within the blink of a watch. If surgical operation is suggested, whether most important or minor, then the optometrist honestly advises the patient approximately the process and sets a date.

All these strategies are short and handy, however they price a hell of quite a few cash. And that's not something many humans can come up with the money for in this stricken economic system, particularly while you take the issue of 'perpetual' lifelong eye care into consideration.

This trouble of lifelong eye care pops up because of the tendency of optometrists to now not offer preventive measures for eye issues.

The hassle with medicinal drug, surgical procedure and optical aids is that they don't cope with the root cause of your eye problems.

You can put on the most powerful prescription eyeglasses or adopt laser surgical treatment to get perfect 20/20 vision once again, however to be able to be for naught if you preserve staring at a computer display all day and fail to relax your eyes in the system. The common person should discover ways to both loosen up and fortify their eyes that allows you to prevent their conditions from worsening in the future.

And in the end, there is the tendency of mainstream docs to be dismissive of alternative strategies of treating issues and sicknesses.

There are very actual gains to be made with alternative remedy, both for illnesses of the eyes, and with illnesses that affect the rest of the body. Sure, there are quacks obtainable who take advantage of people, however there are numerous different opportunity practitioners who have helped cure countless sufferers in their ailments whilst mainstream medicine failed them.

The trouble here is that many mainstream doctors lump all alternative practices with the shams, and outright disregard all other kinds of remedy. This is mainly genuine in specialised niches which include eye care. The average optometrist will only take delivery of his method of treatment as effective. Nothing else works – even when the reasoning in the back of it's far sound, even when endless humans are shouting of its blessings from the rooftops.

Looking at all the problems with mainstream optometry, you can't assist however ask your self: wherein does NVI match in with all this?

Simple: Natural Vision Improvement is an alternative remedy technique that works aspect-through-aspect with mainstream optometry. In fact, it complements the weaknesses of mainstream optometry.

First off is the difficulty of cash.

Many – if now not all – of NVI's activities, exercises and regimens practically fee not anything from your pocket. The easy acts of specializing in a step by step distant object or draping a groovy towel over your eyes value nothing. The activities will then can help you heal and take better care of your eyes without having to spend money for each step of the recovery method.

Now don't take this concept the incorrect way. It is still really worth your money and time to visit your optometrist and are searching for his/her expert opinion on what's incorrect along with your eyes – specifically if you could have enough money it within the first vicinity. But with NVI, at the least you may have an opportunity technique of treatment that does not pressure you to shop for extraordinary instruments or bottles of dubious 'herbal' medicines. You can make the gadgets and prepare the meals by way of yourself (greater on that later in this manual).

NVI will value you next to nothing. Imagine how a whole lot money you would store in case you in no way had to shop for some other pair of glasses or contacts once more.

Next we've the issue of preventive remedy.

NVI isn't always about without delay curing your eye issues with surgery, capsules or optical aids. It is set slowly however gradually improving your potential to see even as developing behavior that prevent further damage on your eyesight. This now not only allows you recover quicker out of your eye problems, but additionally enables prevent future eye troubles as nicely.

Just because we put on glasses, pop a tablet, follow eye drops or adopt surgical procedure does now not mean our eyes are going to be flawlessly first-class.

Many of the problems that have an effect on our vision have a tendency to get worse if we don't provide our eyes the rest and schooling they want.

Even the easy act of analyzing this ebook on a vivid laptop screen for greater than ten mins at a time can put stress to your eyes. If you have been analyzing straight from the creation to this e book, then there is a good danger that you are feeling a stupid ache at the back of your eyes, that the letters are starting to get jumbled up and that it takes extra attempt to make out the man or woman phrases in each line. All of these reactions are signs that your eyes are having trouble reading this text and that you haven't been following the ten-twenty rule – one of many practices that assist save you further damage on your eyes.

And then there's the problem about medical doctors now not accepting any sort of opportunity approach of remedy.

NVI become in no way intended to be a replacement for traditional optometry. Its predecessors – maximum considerably Dr Bates – have been adamant about rejecting optometry. Bates even went up to now as to say glasses do greater harm than good! But the factor about NVI is that it does now not reject traditional understanding. NVI is set applying strategies and exercises that fill within the void of what conventional optometry fails to cope with.

This basically method that NVI's position is to be a associate to traditional optometry. The exercises, activities, regimens and nutritional modifications protected in the NVI software can work to strengthen your eyes, even as conventional optometry deals with the maximum on the spot trouble of being able to see proper now, so that you can drive home and study for your smartphone or laptop.

So wear your glasses at the same time as driving or walking down the road, after which conduct NVI sports inside the protection of your home. Apply the prescribed eye drops in the course of peak hours at the office, then use a chilly towel alternatively when matters calm down. Keep this up, and you may no longer simplest improve your vision but you will also save you your eyes from struggling greater damage than they already have.

So, to wrap up this bankruptcy, Natural Vision Improvement is a modern set of activities that allow you to slowly enhance your eyesight. It isn't always an overnight miracle remedy and it's miles most really not a alternative for optometry, but it IS powerful at a) minimizing damage to your eyes from misuse, b) growing the muscle tissues for your eyes, c) education you to see matters higher and d) imparting your eyes with the vitamins they want to stay robust.

Now that we've mentioned the position of NVI in mainstream optometry, it is time that we delve into every other crucial discussion – expertise how our eyes paintings.

Chapter 2: Understanding How The Eyes Work

Don't fear – I won't proportion a mind-boggling breakdown of the attention's anatomy in this segment. There are sufficient encyclopedic tomes available which might be higher perfect to do that.

What I am going to talk approximately, but, are the components of the eyes which can be immediately inspired, relaxed and/or developed throughout the entire NVI procedure.

Let's begin with the outer, middle and inner layers of the eyes.

The Layers of the Eyes

The outer layer of the eyes is the protecting layer of the eyes.

The massive, milky-white bulk that you see is called the sclera, and that transparent movie that coats the frontal section of the eyeball is the cornea. The cornea is the huge, transparent bulge inside the frontal segment of your eyes. It shields the greater delicate additives of the eye from dust, dirt and other nasty stuff. It is likewise accountable for refracting (bending) a number of the light that hits the eye to create a clearer, greater concise photo. It is one of the maximum touchy tissues in the frame, forcing the muscles of the eyelids shut whilst it is the slightest bit indignant.

The middle layer is wherein a variety of the sensitive components of the eyes are located: the iris, the student, the lens and the ciliary muscle.

The iris is that this round muscle surrounding the scholar, that is the hollow where light passes through. The coloration of the iris varies from man or woman to man or woman, but it's far the contraction of the iris that affects how plenty light gets through to the receptors at the back of the eyes.

The lens is this residue of tissue that focuses light even in addition to provide an accurate image. If you are younger — or have skilled your eyes properly - then the ciliary muscle can be capable of settlement or amplify the lens to consciousness better on an item you want to peer.

And then you definately have the inner layer, which consists of vitreous humor and the retina.

The vitreous humor is that this obvious, gelatinous goop that nourishes the alternative components of the eyes and lets in the eyes to maintain their form. It also features like some thing of a shock absorber so your eyes don't crumble while you get smacked inside the head (or within the eyes).

The retina is wherein all the magic takes place. It consists of the sensitive photoreceptors that remodel mild into indicators that the brain can interpret as snap shots.

This is a short and grimy outline of the extra well-known elements of the eyes, and may be without difficulty determined in basic textbooks at the anatomy of the attention. Keep those components in mind and also you'll see what precise part of the attention our later sports and regimens will recognition on. Now allow's circulate directly to how we use our eyes.

Central Vision

When you need to take a look at one precise factor, you consciousness your eyes to higher see some thing it's miles you need to have a look at. This kind of imaginative and prescient is referred to as valuable imaginative and prescient, additionally referred to as foveal vision. This sort of 'seeing' helps you to cognizance your attention on a novel object as well as close by things surrounding the point of interest of your interest.

Central imaginative and prescient is also called foveal imaginative and prescient due to the fact the a part of the eye that makes this possible is called the fovea centralis.

The fovea centralis (or actually the fovea) is filled with small, dense photoreceptors that turn light into electric powered signals. The hassle with the fovea, but, is that it's far not able to receive enough blood whilst uncovered to bright light. This can even attain the factor of hypoxia, wherein the cells within the fovea die if they may be exposed to light that is too brilliant. Remember the ten-twenty rule? This is why I recommend which you prevent every ten mins and look away for twenty seconds at the same time as reading this ebook – especially if you're studying it off a computer screen and extra-so in case you are analyzing the tiny letters to your cellphone.

Improving valuable vision is one of the leader aims of Natural Vision Improvement. Training the muscular tissues of the eyes – from the iris to the ciliary muscle – will let you see higher from a physiological factor of view. Training your mind to better interpret the alerts received from the fovea will let you see better from a neurological factor of view. Combine the two together and also you'll be higher able to concentrate on what you need to peer.

Peripheral Vision

If primary vision is all approximately that specialize in one precise issue, then peripheral vision includes being privy to the whole lot that your eyes can see. Peripheral imaginative and prescient is some thing that most people take for granted, but becoming ignorant of the things we don't cognizance on can be simply as crippling as losing our potential to focus on one issue.

Good peripheral imaginative and prescient is something that takes a number of exercise and training to grasp. This is because of the subjective position of awareness. We regularly pass by way of the day ignoring the entirety around us and focusing simplest on what we want to do. This is not the case for certain people like jugglers, chess masters or real-time strategy sport (RTS) players.

Jugglers teach themselves to be aware about the place of the items they're juggling, which is critical due to the fact they can not cognizance on just one item at a time.

Chess masters need to be completely aware about all the pieces at the board. RTS players want to do the identical with their games, despite the fact that the glare from the TV or laptop display will likely do extra damage than good for their standard imaginative and prescient.

Certain sports in Natural Vision Improvement also purpose to increase your peripheral vision on the identical time as your relevant imaginative and prescient. After all, you would possibly need to peer that rushing car, that sparking outlet or that precariously-positioned toddler even whilst you don't cognizance your eyesight on them.

Now that we've long gone over the fundamental components of the eyes and the two ways we use our eyes to look the sector round us, it's time we were given down to the meat and bones of this manual: the real processes concerned in Natural Vision Improvement. Let's begin with the perfect ones – sports that help loosen up the eyes.

NVI EYE RELAXATION ACTIVITIES

One of the primary motives the eyes have a tendency to fail through the years is because of excessive strain. We often take our eyes with no consideration; abusing them to the factor in which they start bogging down and failing on us. This is in particular authentic in the current day.

We live within the facts and virtual amusement age, wherein we glue our eyes to the laptop and TV displays for hours on cease every day. It doesn't matter whether or not you're a younger technophile dabbling in the modern-day and greatest video game or a hectic 50-something retaining tabs at the state-of-the-art traits on Wall Street – chances are you are the use of your eyes an excessive amount of and in the wrong way. We truely can't live in modern-day society if we dispose of our digital monitors—computers, TVs, clever phones, e-readers and capsules.

But we are able to provide our eyes sufficient time to rest and get over the punishment we heap upon them on a ordinary basis. Here are a number of the sports to help you do simply that:

The 'Ten-Twenty' Rule

One of the maximum essential things you may do to save you damage on your eyes is to in reality look far from your laptop display screen now and again.

1. Prepare a timer. You can buy one out of your nearby department shop or you could download an app from the Internet. I use one referred to as "Tomato One" on my Mac.

2. Set it to head off each ten mins before you start working or analyzing.

three. Every time the timer goes off, stop searching at your laptop display and look at some thing else within the room for 20 seconds – preferably out your window if you could.

Why do you want to try this? Well, we have a tendency to forget about to blink when we're deeply engrossed in some thing that includes the usage of our eyes. This is specially actual while we are analyzing or the use of a computer screen.

This unconscious act of no longer blinking irritates our eyes due to the fact the tears that must coat the eyeball are not spread round. The tears stay installed one region, so the eyes get lots more strained than they ought to be.

The act of searching away also does every other aspect – it offers the muscular tissues within the eyes a while to relaxation. Not only do our eyes dry out if we don't blink often enough, however the sheer fatigue of focusing our eyes for prolonged intervals of time can do some severe damage over time.

Taking your eyes off the display every ten minutes or so, takes away the tension from your eye muscle tissues, stopping any in addition deterioration on your vision.

It allows to know that so one can focus on something close by (like a ebook or a pc screen), the ciliary muscle needs to be in a shrunk state so that it can make the jelly lens to your eye fatter. This fattening of the lens is what lets in mild coming from a nearby supply, to be nicely targeted. Maintaining this for a long term ends in eye stress, and it's far widely recognized that eye stress is the primary motive of bad and deteriorating eyesight.

Here's a bit test you may do to verify this.

Hold the palm of your give up your face, touching the bridge of your nostril. With your hand held this close, try to consciousness your eyes at the lines for your palm. You will locate that you may't cognizance your eyes and get a clean view, because your hand is too near and your jelly lens simply can't get fats enough.

Now, slowly pass your hand away from your eyes till you may reap clean cognizance. This will show up approximately an inch or two away from your eyes. Now maintain this attention for so long as you may. Notice how a great deal pressure it causes on your eyes to maintain this awareness. This is because at this factor, your ciliary muscle, and different eye muscle mass involved in lodging, are at maximal contraction.

Conversely, do you bear in mind the ultimate time you were having a pipe dream? Was there any strain in any way for your eyes at the same time as you have been in that trance? Well of path no longer. When you are daydreaming your eyes are absolutely defocused. The ciliary muscle for your eye is absolutely relaxed, so there is no construct-up of eye strain. Focusing on a distance object with the aid of looking at distant gadgets in your room, or maybe better, searching out the window, has a comparable effect. In order to awareness light from distant gadgets, the jelly lens in your eye has to come to be lengthy and flat. This is performed by way of enjoyable the ciliary muscle.

A variation of the 'ten-twenty' rule is the 'thirty-sixty' rule. If you without a doubt want to concentrate for prolonged periods of time, then set your timer to go off each thirty minutes rather than ten. The trap is which you need to rest your eyes for a complete minute. Get up, stretch a piece, cross for a drink of water – sixty seconds is a huge window to transport your frame a bit even as resting your eyes at the identical time.

Interval Reading

If you do a whole lot of studying in your process, studies or enjoyment time, then you will locate c language studying to be a pretty useful little tool to lessen the pressure for your eyes:

1. When studying, awareness your attention to the empty spaces in between the strains of textual content. Do NOT read the text itself. Read in a consistent left-right sweeping movement transferring one line down as you finish reading every line.

2. Practice c program languageperiod reading till you could effortlessly make out the phrases in each line.

The most not unusual technique of reading is to take a look at the words. The problem with this technique of reading is the high assessment of the black text on the plain — and regularly white — history. We for this reason consciousness our relevant imaginative and prescient on black letters against a completely shiny and empty historical past; inflicting a tremendous amount of strain to our eyes within the manner.

The simple act of moving your central imaginative and prescient to the brilliant and empty background can clearly remove numerous that strain. This is due to the fact the iris and the fovea centralis alter to the a lot extra considerable white historical past as opposed to the smaller, greater complex black letters. Our brains can fill within the blanks, so to talk, to form words and sentences although we don't attention solely at the text.

You could even locate yourself studying quicker in case you grasp c program languageperiod analyzing. You will find your self spending less time focusing on the letters as you better utilize your thoughts to interpret the meaning in the back of the aggregate of letters and numbers in whatever you're studying.

Touch Typing

This one is pretty easy: learn how to type while not having to take a look at the keyboard or the screen. You can take contact typing classes or download programs that train you a way to kind better – whatever will work so long as you are capable of grasp the skill.

Now what does contact typing have to do with relaxing your eyes? Well, you may work to your pc without having to have a look at the display the whole time. If you're a professional touch typist, then you could near your eyes for multiple seconds - even a couple of minutes - even as typing out what you want to type out. This easy act of remaining your eyes every few seconds or so can help decrease the strain on your eyes.

And it additionally enables which you get matters finished faster. The less time spent typing and staring at the screen, the better to your eyes.

Back once I turned into in university, I took a touch typing direction on the aspect for just one hour a week. At first once I tried to touch kind, I changed into typing at a snail-pace compared to my preceding typing pace and as compared to all people round me. However, after some months, I changed into typing quicker than anybody I knew, AND I should do it with my eyes closed!

Since then, that one hour a week I invested has paid again masses of times over, in all the time I actually have stored with my newfound light-speed typing.

So, if you spend any time in the front of a laptop, I enormously suggest you make investments the time to discover ways to touch-type. Not only due to the fact it may assist save your eyes when you type occasionally along with your eyes closed, however additionally because you may make that point lower back and more with quicker typing abilities.

Another alternative is to put money into dictation software, the likes of Dragon Naturally Speaking. These may be very annoying to paintings with before everything, however after you've learned all the little instructions and shortcuts, you'll end up saving your eyes and saving an entire bunch of time.

Eye Washing

One of the greater soothing solutions to help relax your eyes after a long day's work is to immediately wash your eyes with a water solution. This is in particular vital for folks who stay in dry environments in which there are a whole lot of unfastened-floating particles of dust or dust, like city and industrial environments.

1. Pour one drop of freshly squeezed lemon juice into a cup of lukewarm distilled water. Mix the solution properly. Prepare spare cups of distilled lukewarm water if this is the primary time you are attempting the answer.

2. Take a remedy dropper and use it to generously practice a couple of drops of the solution to each eye. Let the solution run out of your eyes. You might also want to use a towel to seize the runoff.

three. Keep making use of the answer and alternating between every eye till the cup is empty. Do this day by day for one week. If your eyes are excessively angry and stay indignant for 5 mins after making use of the answer, use the cup of lukewarm distilled water to clean out the answer.

4. If you sense no damaging outcomes from the answer, then boom its potency via using two drops of lemon juice rather than just one after the first week. Move on to three drops after the 0.33 week and upload no greater than that.

This solution is used commonly to cleanse and reduce inflammation inside the eyes after regular exposure to dust, dust, smoke and other pollution that we're exposed to in modern society.

There is the possibility, however, that your eyes can be touchy to even this diluted answer of lemon juice. If this occurs to you, then virtually use natural distilled lukewarm water instead. It is not as mighty as the lemon solution, however as a minimum you're nevertheless bodily washing out the particles that get stuck on your eyes.

Note that it's vital to apply only distilled water, not filtered water, and really not tap water. Distilled water is the simplest form of purified water that has all micro organism and viruses removed from it. Even the quality form of water filtration—opposite osmosis— can let bacteria and viruses through to the water.

Cool Towels

If you're busy at paintings and locate that your eyes are becoming mainly tired, then all you want to do is run a few high-quality, cool tap water on a small face towel and allow it drape across your closed eyes for a couple of minutes.

You can't get a greater easy NVI eye rest technique than that.

The soothing results of water can help relax your eyes after consistent use, that is specially important for the busy office employee who cannot keep away from watching a laptop display for hours on cease. Not handiest will this relax your eyes, however it may additionally assist de-strain you at the identical time. Simply leaning returned towards your chair, resting your head lower back and simply closing your eyes for a few minutes can do wonders for you within the workplace.

Hot and Cold Towels

While cool towels are a short and convenient way to loosen up your eyes at the same time as at work, you could in reality use the restorative outcomes of hot and bloodless towels to assist heal your eyes whilst at domestic.

1. Prepare the following: a basin of steaming (now not boiling) warm water, a basin of ice-bloodless water and two small face towels. I would propose doing this rest exercising within the tub if feasible, it's simply less complicated that manner.

2. Dip one face towel into the basin containing warm water. Wring out the water and drape the nevertheless-warm face towel over your closed eyes. Do this for 30 seconds. Be cautious of spilling water in case you aren't inside the bath.

three. Remove the recent towel from your eyes and place it inside the hot water basin. Take the other face towel and dip into the basin containing ice-bloodless water. Drape this towel over your closed eyes for 30 seconds.

4. Alternate among the recent and bloodless cycle 7 times.

Now the purpose behind alternating between hot and cold water is to promote blood drift in and across the eyes. The heat pulls in blood from the body in an try and cool off the heated areas, at the same time as the bloodless reasons the frame to pull blood faraway from that area to preserve warmth.

Promoting better blood flow in and around the eyes does very critical things:

1. It permits the blood to higher bring in oxygen and vitamins that nourish the cells in the eyes.

2. It permits the blood to are available and eliminate the lifeless and damaged cells inside the eyes.

This is also a completely vital hobby if you hold on staring at the brilliant display screen of a computer all day lengthy. Remember the thing about the cells inside the fovea centralis – the part of the attention devoted to significant imaginative and prescient – loss of life off from overexposure to light? Using the recent and bloodless remedy need to help your eyes better cope with the aftereffects of this regular publicity to light from a pc display screen.

Sunning

Yes, looking immediately on the solar is bad and can permanently harm your eyes, however the rays of the solar however play an important position in both your eyesight and your normal fitness.

1. Choose a time maximum convenient for you: from sunrise up to 10am or from 3pm up to dusk.

2. Find a spot wherein you could get plenty of sunshine. Sit down in that spot even as letting your complete body relax

three. Look on the sky at an perspective wherein you get some sunlight shining for your face with out searching at once on the sun.

4. Slowly swing your head to and fro for 2 to three mins. Make positive you do not appearance without delay at the sun. Blink a few times once in a while to unfold some tears over your eyes.

**In addition to everyday sunning, ensure which you get as a minimum two to a few hours of herbal publicity to the solar every day. Your eyes ought to at the least get a healthful dose of indirect sunlight for two to 3 hours an afternoon.

The primary reason of this hobby is to expose your eyes to the warmth of the solar when it's far at its gentlest – from sunrise to 10am and from 3pm to nightfall. These are the instances whilst the sun isn't throwing out insane quantities of ultraviolet rays and as a substitute promises a softer, greater relaxing dose of diet D to the frame.

The modern day studies are showing that vitamin D is much less of a diet and extra of a hormone, with wide-ranging fitness blessings, from supporting you to resist disorder, to broaden stronger bones, shed pounds, fight despair, fatigue, and more. Vitamin D also helps save you and reverse age-associated eyesight deterioration by way of removing the build-up of particles and poisonous deposits from the tiniest capillaries that supply blood to your eyes.

The solar's rays can nourish your eyes and enhance your imaginative and prescient, however they also can be damaging. To avoid any harm, never look at once on the solar, and try to avoid the solar from the hours of

10am to 3pm, while the sun's UV rays are at their most powerful.

Take for instance a look at accomplished on college leavers in Asian towns as reported by means of the BBC. These youngsters spend a lot time interior studying, looking TV, or gambling video video games, that their eyes certainly elongate and turn out to be quick-sighted. The researchers in the back of the observe be aware that the shortage of exposure to daylight performs a chief function in their brief-sightedness, that's why they suggest youngsters get at least to a few hours of sunlight each day.

Face and Neck Massage

The face and neck include quite a few muscular tissues which can be hotspots for pressure buildup. This is why your head and neck hurt plenty whilst you are going via intervals of extreme stress – stress that may in the end spill over for your eyes and affect your eyesight if left unchecked.

The great thing you may do is to visit a professional rub down parlor and time table normal classes on a weekly foundation. You can also massage your very own face and neck for the ones long, stressful days through following these simple steps to conduct your own mini self-rub down habitual:

1. Begin through rubbing your palms softly but firmly in opposition to every different. This builds up heat so one can be used later at some point of the rubdown.

2. Close your eyes and lightly rub the temples of your head with your palms. Do this for approximately ten to fifteen seconds.

three. Move right down to the joints of the jaw just underneath the ears and lightly rub them with your palms. Do this for another ten to fifteen seconds.

four. Now use your thumbs to softly stroke your eyebrows outwards from the pinnacle of the bridge of your nostril. Another ten to fifteen seconds need to suffice.

five. Use your index and center arms to gently stroke the vicinity underneath the eyes; tracing the edge of the bone as you achieve this. Ten to fifteen seconds all over again.

6. Rub your arms softly however firmly again before proceeding.

7. Turn your head to the proper and sense the muscle that runs down from the ear on your neck. It need to protrude when turning. Use the hands of your right hand to gently palpate or periodically practice pressure to this muscle. Do this for ten to 15 seconds earlier than repeating the complete process – this time turning to the left and the use of your left hand to palpate the muscle.

8. Now attain up with both hands and locate the muscle tissues around the returned of your neck. Gently practice strain along with your hands; leading right down to the bottom of the neck near the shoulders for some other ten to fifteen seconds.

9. Finally, slowly twist your neck to one facet while looking to attain your chin to your shoulder. You have to sense a moderate pull on your neck if performed efficiently. Do this about 5 instances for every facet and you ought to be performed along with your mini self-massage habitual.

Now recall that the entire point of this interest is to lessen the pent-up anxiety simply around the eyes. It may not appear relevant to relaxing your eyes, but the anxiety within the neck and face regions can ultimately affect your eyesight – in particular after a long day's work at the workplace.

And except, you can observe up your face and neck rub down with a extra direct eye rub down: palming.

Palming

While it's usually not an excellent concept to without delay rub our eyes and threat exposing them to blunt trauma, it IS a very good idea to enhance blood go with the flow to your eyes. This is where palming is available in.

1. Wash your arms with soap and water. Dry them thoroughly afterwards.

2. Rub your arms gently but firmly together till they are as warm as you can cope with.

3. Dim the lighting for your room. Close your eyes and lay the nevertheless-warm hands of your fingers on them. Cup your eyes as you do

so and ensure that you surround your eye socket with the palm of your hand.

four. Now simply take a seat again, relax and lighten up your whole frame – in particular the muscle groups in and around your face.

five. Visualize smooth, easy and velvet black. Breath as slowly, gently and softly as you may without straining your lungs.

6. [Optional step] Slowly and emphatically repeat the phrase "I see well" with each exhaling breath.

7. Keep this up for 5 to fifteen minutes or longer.

8. Lift your palms out of your face and slowly open your eyes. Blink a few times to regulate to the light, which need to be less complicated if you dimmed the lighting fixtures.

The whole point of palming is fourfold:

1. To relax your eyes whilst draining out the tension.

2. To promote better blood stream by means of exposing the eyes to warmth from the hands.

3. To relax your thoughts, thereby enhancing the thoughts-eye connection, and also enhancing the translation of snap shots with the aid of your brain.

four. To encourage you to keep pursuing better imaginative and prescient.

The last point is particularly critical. Most human beings are straitjacketed into believing that there's no manner they are able to see higher without their glasses or steeply-priced surgery. Encouraging your self has no tangible and instantaneous benefits for your eyesight, however it does help hold your spirits up alongside the complete method. This high-quality method additionally has beneficial results within the "seeing" exercises within the following bankruptcy.

There is extra to palming than just setting your fingers over your eyes. The secret lies in reaching a deep country of relaxation.

When palming, do recollect not to nod off. Contrary to popular notion, your eyes are not all that relaxed while drowsing. 20-25% of overall sleep time in adults is spent in speedy eye motion (REM) sleep. During REM sleep, you're all but relaxed. Not handiest are your eyes shifting swiftly and randomly, but your brain pastime increases, your coronary heart price is going up, and your respiratory gets quicker.

Through palming and meditation (mentioned under), you may reap far deeper levels of rest than through sleep.

"Emptying" Meditation

I cannot emphasize the significance of rest sufficient, and meditation is one of the key approaches you can break out from worldly concerns for some precious moments before coming lower back to the awful fact of lifestyles.

Palming is a mild shape of meditation, although the focal point on your eyes does dilute the 'emptying' experience of meditation. This is why you still need to meditate and visualize vacancy to completely get rid of the pressure which you have built up over the day:

1. Find a comfortable region to sit down down. You do no longer need to get into the classical lotus function to meditate. The best component that subjects is which you are comfortable and able to sit along with your back instantly to facilitate true respiration.

2. Relax your body. Tilt your head down slightly and permit your fingers drop down loose. You can rest your fingers to your thighs or you can allow them to grasp freely on the sides.

three. Focus only on deep, slow and solemn breathing. Breathe inside and outside as deeply as you can tolerate without feeling any pain. Think of nothing else besides your respiration. If executed successfully, you must sense an uplifting sensation with every breath.

4. Once you set up your rhythm of respiratory and might effects breathe deeply without questioning an excessive amount of approximately it, the next element you want to do is to clean all mind out of your mind.

You can start this with the aid of counting your breaths from one to ten and then going back to one. You also can prefer to repeat a chain of words – mantras – with each exhale. Doing so will awareness your mind faraway from outside distractions and pull them in the direction of an 'empty' nation of thoughts.

five. Maintain the 'empty' state of mind for as long as possible. Meditating is great performed if you have no upcoming engagements so you don't need to reflect onconsideration on anything. Meditating just earlier than going to sleep is a splendid pastime to help you de-pressure earlier than tucking in for the night time.

Meditation is the top of all relaxation sports even supposing it isn't always manifestly associated with the eyes at first look. As I've referred to typically earlier than, the collecting stress in our lives has a way of seeping into and tensing up the muscle mass that immediately have an effect on our eyes. This tension can then devour away on the eyes until your vision begins to go to pot.

And except, pressure performs an excellent larger position in lifestyles in fashionable. Being constantly frustrated, irritable and combative all of the time isn't a great way to enjoy life.

Chapter 3: Nvi "Seeing" Exercises

Now that you have a few eye rest physical activities below your belt, you are geared up to begin schooling your eyes to paintings and see matters better.

An vital note before analyzing through this chapter: DO NOT OVERSTRAIN YOUR EYES! I will listing down the precise schooling exercises right here, but it's miles critical that you take everything slow & constant. Later in this ebook I will give you a weekly regimen for each rest activities and seeing sporting events, so simply take a seat tight and get yourself up to speed with the sporting activities before going all out and seeking to repair your imaginative and prescient in a single exercising :) .

Oh, and one greater issue – TAKE OFF YOUR GLASSES WHILE CONDUCTING ALL OF THESE 'SEEING' EXERCISES! You need to teach your eyes to see higher on their own, so set apart your glasses whilst you train.

Power Eye Stretches

One of the first and easiest matters you may do to directly improve your eyesight is to reinforce the muscle groups that manipulate the movement of your eyeballs.

1. Start by means of setting up a chair for your room. Place an item like a photo body or a clock about six ft away from you. Make positive it is placed on a flat, solid surface.

2. Now near your left eye and squeeze your eyelid close as hard as you could control with out inflicting pain. Make certain that your eyelids don't pucker out while you do this, otherwise you risk scratching or abrading the sensitive skin below it.

3. Maintain this squeeze for ten seconds. Close your eyes and allow your eyes relaxation for the identical quantity of time.

4. Repeat this squeeze for another ten seconds together with your proper eye. Close and relaxation your eyes for every other ten seconds.

five. Now squeeze down difficult with each eyes close tight accompanied by means of ten seconds of relaxation.

6. Now orient your face in the direction of the item you positioned in the front of you. Look as difficult as you could to the left with both eyes even as nonetheless keeping your face orientated toward the object in the front of you. Close and rest your eyes for ten seconds.

7. Repeat the previous manner, this time looking as difficult as you may to the proper with out shifting your head.

8. Repeat the technique looking up and then searching down with your eyes. Remember to relax and close them after looking hard in any path.

nine. Once all corners were given 'electricity' stretches, wind down by means of palming your eyes. Refer to the previous bankruptcy on the way to well palm your eyes.

The entire purpose of power eye stretches is to bolster the muscular tissues that control the motion of your eyeballs. This is an vital first step within the Natural Vision Improvement manner because it builds a strong muscular basis to your eyes as a way to pass around with less effort and much less stress.

Focus Training

One of the most simple techniques of sharpening your eyesight is to teach the muscle tissue that are chargeable for specializing in objects of varying distances.

1. Start via pinpointing a far off object that is extra than 30 toes far from your modern area. While it's far most popular which you search for a tree, mountain, shrub or a few different natural item to look at (for the calming impact nature has on us), any distant item like a automobile or constructing will do for this workout.

2. Now put together a small piece of stiff paper or card. Write down a chain of letters on that piece of paper. Make certain the lettering is massive sufficient with a view to easily apprehend at arm's duration.

3. Start by masking your proper eye along with your proper hand at the same time as using your left hand to keep the small piece of paper upright at arm's period, with the letters facing you. Align the paper just beside the remote item you have pinpointed. Take 5

seconds to attention and pick out each individual letter written on the piece of paper.

four. Now take a look at the remote item for five seconds. While you are doing so, pass the piece of paper an inch toward you.

5. Shift your attention returned to the paper. Focus and become aware of the letters once again.

6. Repeat the technique from step four; transferring the paper closer and nearer until your eye gets tired or the letters are too near your face to nicely pick out.

7. Now repeat the entire manner starting from step three – this time overlaying your left eye at the same time as switching fingers.

8. Repeat the whole method once again while maintaining each eyes open. Use any hand you prefer to hold the cardboard upright.

** Remember to attention at the shape, size and details of every letter at the piece of paper. Simply spotting the letters will now not educate your eyes to better consciousness.

This complete manner goals to train your eyes to higher cognizance at objects that get steadily closer on your vision. Remember how the ciliary muscle adjusts the lens? This pastime will teach your ciliary muscle tissue to better adapt to regularly closer gadgets and is specifically beneficial for farsighted people (although it's very effective for nearsighted people too). It is a important aspect of Natural Vision Improvement training, so don't skip out on it even supposing you could without problems see things near you.

Distance Focus Training

But what approximately steadily distant objects? This is wherein distance recognition training comes into the picture.

1. Start via pinpointing a series of remote objects that step by step get further and similarly far from your current region. For example, you may word a stop sign 20 ft away, a parked automobile 30 feet away, a comfort store signal 40 ft away after which a site visitors light 60 toes away (even though

herbal gadgets could be higher — e.G. Timber planted at unique distances).

2. Prepare a small piece of stiff paper or card. Write down a sequence of letters on that piece of paper. Make sure the lettering is big enough in an effort to effortlessly recognize at arm's period.

three. Start through protecting your right eye with your right hand even as the use of your left hand to keep the small piece of paper upright with the letters facing you. Align this piece of paper just beside the closest remote object you have got pinpointed. Focus and identify every person letter written on the piece of paper.

four. Now in preference to bringing the card toward you, hold that card at arm's duration even as shifting your imaginative and prescient toward the progressively in addition objects. In our example, you must awareness your attention to the stop sign for ten seconds, then the letters on the card, then the parked car, back to the letters, then the ease keep sign, lower back to the letters once more, then the traffic mild and sooner or later again to the letters.

five. Now repeat the complete system beginning from step 3 – this time overlaying your left eye even as switching palms.

6. Repeat the whole procedure yet again even as retaining each eyes open. Use any hand you favor to preserve the cardboard upright.

** Remember to cognizance on the form, length and info of each letter at the piece of paper, and additionally of the objects in the distance. Simply recognizing the letters and items will now not educate your eyes to higher consciousness.

Distance recognition schooling develops your ciliary muscle tissues to better modify to regularly remote gadgets. This is an particularly useful exercising for folks who are nearsighted (myopic), as they have the most problem focusing on remote objects without the aid of glasses. Still, distance attention education is something that everybody seeking to reinforce his or her vision needs to do to be able to create a balanced routine.

Tracing

Tracing is a supplementary exercising to distance focusing, which similarly develops your capacity to peer distant objects clearer and with better acuity. This is beneficial for both close to and farsighted individuals, mainly in terms of growing telescopic imaginative and prescient – being capable of see remote items with more readability.

1. Purchase or make your very own Snellen eye chart. You can locate a proof and a few printable Snellen eye charts on https://www.Disabled-world.Com/calculators-charts/snellen-charts.Php. You'll also discover loose printable Snellen charts in the appendix portion on the stop of this ebook.

2. Pin the Snellen eye chart at the wall. Stand 10 ft away and recognition at the smallest possible letters that you may see with out your glasses.

three. Now choose one letter and follow its outline along with your eyes, 'tracing' it with as an awful lot depth and electricity as you could muster with out hurting your eyes.

4. Close your eyes for 5 seconds and hint the letter another time. Remember to accomplish that with energy and depth.

5. Close your eyes a 2d time and 'palm' them. Refer to the previous chapter on a way to palm your eyes.

6. Visualize the define of the letter even as palming your eyes.

7. Exhale whilst opening your eyes and consciousness over again at the letter. It need to become a piece clearer now, or at the very least seem darker than earlier than.

8. Keep looking at the letter while slowly, very slowly, swaying from side to side.

nine. After some seconds of swaying, take one quick step backwards. Step backwards some more until you may no longer apprehend the letter. Stop straight away at this point.

10. Now bend ahead until you can make out the letter over again. If you can't make out the letter whilst bending forward, take one brief leap forward till you could see the letter while bending.

eleven. Now slowly straighten your back and focus on the letter whilst swaying from side to side.

12. Keep focusing on the letter for approximately ten seconds earlier than repeating the workout for the alternative letters till you whole the whole row of letters at the chart.

The entire factor of this exercising is to regularly enhance your capability to peer distant items with greater readability. This makes tracing, an outstanding complement to the preceding sporting activities designed to better adjust your eyesight to close by gadgets.

Fast Focus Training

The preceding techniques of focus education involved slow, deliberate shifts in attention. This time, you will need to higher understand an object that movements fast between more than one distances.

1. Prepare a card much like the ones used for cognizance schooling and distance attention education.

2. Use your left hand to cowl your left eye at the same time as the usage of your proper hand to keep the cardboard at arm's period.

3. Focus on the letters on the cardboard whilst slowly and gradually bringing it closer to your right eye. Maintain a tempo wherein you could without difficulty understand the letters with out straining your eyes too much.

four. Once the cardboard reaches a distance wherein you may now not recognize the letters on the cardboard, straight away 'whip' the card lower back to arm's period. Focus on the letters as fast and as correctly as you could.

five. Repeat this workout ten instances.

6. Now opposite your arms – proper hand to cover your proper eye whilst the usage of your left hand to deliver the card towards

your left eye. Repeat the exercising ten instances.

7. Repeat the exercise some other ten instances at the same time as using both your eyes. Use your selected arm for this final round.

eight. Now repeat the complete exercise from step 2. This time, reverse the path of the card. Instead of slowly bringing the cardboard to you, slowly deliver the card far from you whilst 'whipping' it just a few inches far from your face. Be careful no longer to strike yourself at the same time as doing so.

The factor of this training exercising is to higher alter your eyes to rapid-moving items that trade distances in the blink of an eye. Remember to recognition on all of the details of the letters on the cardboard instead of really spotting them.

Peripheral Gazing

All the activities to date are designed to enhance your principal vision – your capability to recognition on one precise item at a time. Peripheral staring at will teach your capacity to better understand things even whilst you aren't specially looking at them.

1. Prepare bright yellow pencils. Hold them upright at eye degree, about six inches apart and twelve inches from your face.

2. For the whole duration of this exercise, you will cognizance your relevant imaginative and prescient on an object inside the distance, in among the pencils. At the same time, without searching directly at either pencil (i.E. By means of the use of your peripheral vision), attempt to observe each element you may about the yellow pencils.

three. Now, slowly move the pencils far from each other till you could slightly see them along with your peripheral vision. Keep your awareness locked on that distant item.

four. Slowly pull lower back the pencils till they may be six inches aside from every other again. Repeat from step 2 for a complete of ten instances.

five. Now flow one pencil upwards and the other downwards till you could no longer see them along with your peripheral imaginative and prescient. Once this occurs, reverse the motion of every pencil. Repeat ten instances – 5 instances in a single route, five times the other.

6. Now you want to move the pencils diagonally. Center your pencils to eye degree. Move the right pencil upward and to the right at the same time as shifting the left pencil downward and to the left.

7. Once you can now not see the pencils, slowly circulate them back to the center. This time you'll circulate your right pencil downward and to the right at the same time as shifting the left pencil upward and to the left.

8. Repeat steps five and six for a complete of ten instances – 5 for one direction and five for the alternative.

nine. Center the pencils to eye stage. Trace circles together with your palms – the left going counterclockwise and the right going clockwise. The circles have to be extensive enough that you may barely see the pencils when they may be furthest away from you. Do this ten times.

10. Now reverse the rotation of the pencils – left going clockwise and right going counterclockwise. Do this for some other ten instances.

The distinct positions of the pencil, blended with its vibrant yellow shade, will higher expand your capability to see things even while you aren't specializing in them in any respect – that is a must in view that many of our cutting-edge-day occupations like workplace work weakens and diminishes our peripheral imaginative and prescient.

Juggling

Believe it or no longer, gaining knowledge of how to juggle is one of the maximum dynamic (not to mention a laugh) approaches you may train your peripheral vision. Here is a brief and smooth guide on the way to juggle everyday tennis balls:

1. Prepare three tennis balls (though juggling balls are higher if you have a hard and fast).

2. Take one tennis ball. Throw it up to eye stage with one hand and use the other hand to capture it. If accomplished efficiently, you

have to form an arc that is approximately eye stage with each throw. Practice until you're capable of trap the ball with minimum effort.

3. Now you may learn how to begin a -ball juggle. Take two tennis balls. First, throw the ball on your right hand to your left hand as outlined in the previous step. Just as this primary ball reaches its maximum point within the arc, throw the ball for your left hand up within the air up for your proper hand. Stop when you efficaciously catch each balls. This is where matters begin to get elaborate. Avoid the urge to honestly pass the ball in your proper hand to your left hand on the nearest point. You should form a watch-level arc as you toss each ball, otherwise you may not be able to juggle 3 balls. Since each balls are going up in an arc, you also should time and intention your throws to prevent the balls from colliding mid-air.

4. Practice the preceding step time and again once more until you're comfortable with the right-left throw. Now switch arms, beginning with your left hand then accompanied by using your proper. Remember, you are not constantly juggling simply but, you are just

beginning a two-ball juggle, and preventing as quickly as one ball has landed in each hand.

5. Once you're able to start a juggle with either hand, practice juggling both balls continuously. The trick is to usually have one hand free, so earlier than the ball lands in one hand, you have to toss the ball inside the different hand inside the air.

6. If you have mastered the previous step, then it's time to throw in the third ball. Start via maintaining two balls together with your dominant hand and one ball along with your off hand. Let's expect you're right passed on this lesson.

7. Throw the primary ball along with your proper hand, so it goes up in an arc, over towards your left hand.

8. Just because the first ball reaches its highest factor, throw the second ball – the only for your left hand – up to your right. Just as this 2d ball reaches its highest factor, throw the alternative ball in your proper hand – the 1/3 ball – to your left hand. This is the trickiest part of the three-ball juggle. You will need to throw-capture-throw-catch-throw-

capture in rapid succession. It takes practice, however you'll quickly get the flow in case you preserve it at it.

nine. Keep repeating the sample and you'll soon be capable of juggle 3 balls like a seasoned.

The factor approximately juggling is that you are pressured to rely upon your peripheral vision instead of your vital vision. Focusing on one ball for too lengthy will reason you to lose sight of the final balls, so that you sharpen you peripheral imaginative and prescient as you master the finer elements of juggling. You may even pass on to more superior juggling techniques – like the half-shower/1/2-arc approach for juggling three balls – if you stick at it lengthy enough.

Juggling goes past simply reaping rewards your eyesight. I for my part have observed juggling to be extraordinarily healing. Not best does it calm and soothe me, it de-stresses my eyes and my thoughts, and even elevates my mood. So I become on no account amazed to research of something referred to as 'juggling therapy' – a whole discipline in itself, based on the premise that juggling contributes to adjustments in emotional memory processing. Studies have observed juggling remedy to be beneficial inside the management of strain and tension.

Unlike other styles of multi-tasking, juggling now not best reduces anxiety and pressure, however it also improves your eyesight and springs with an entire host of other blessings.

Juggling is also associated with progressed eye-hand coordination, physical health, balance, rhythm, and reflexes. Juggling affords you with a far-wished right mind smash in a left-mind dominant world.

As a proper-brain interest, juggling improves your creativity, will increase your visible/spatial intelligence, and usually makes you smarter. And it's now not just hocus-pocus conjecture, scientists have found that juggling simply reasons your brain to generate new synaptic connections, stimulating grey count increase, and making your mind larger.

So as hard and irritating as it is able to be to examine in the beginning, juggling is absolutely one of these competencies that truely is well worth studying.

As defined above, you could use tennis balls, or maybe pieces of lego, however juggling balls are generally simpler to study with, due to the fact they're designed to match properly into your hand, and very importantly, they do not jump and are easy to trap. Learn with juggling balls first to minimise frustration, then you could learn how to juggle with different items.

Chapter 4: Your Nvi Regimen

Now which you understand what the sporting activities and activities are, and how to do them, it's time to match them right into a regimen on your eyes.

Here is a pattern regimen of ways you can observe the formerly discussed exercises on a weekly foundation:

This is a simple and simple regimen that will help you to get began along with your Natural Vision Improvement program. It is likewise perfect for the typical busy present day way of life, as the routine does no longer call for an excessive amount of time for your part. You can alter the routine for your wishes, however simply do not forget no longer to overdo it with the education physical games.

If you like, it is perfectly appropriate to start with simply the relaxation sports. Dr Bates, and lots of NVI therapists that observed (myself protected), strongly believed (and still trust) that relaxation by myself can bring about brilliant enhancements on your vision.

In truth, in lots of instances, the relaxation exercises are all that a trainee wishes.

To ease into this system, begin with just one rest workout like palming. Do it for five-15 minutes daily until you get excellent at it. As you get better at palming, you'll locate that you could set off a kingdom of deep relaxation inside seconds of getting started out.

Once you've got carried out an amazing stage of proficiency with palming, upload in every other workout, then any other and so on. Over time you'll have a repertoire of different sporting activities that you may name upon on every occasion you experience adore it. You will recognise which sporting events work great for you, and you may assemble your personal regimen that you're feeling works great in your very own personal needs.

Change is a completely tough component. People generally seem to be hell-bent towards it, that is why most people find it not possible to lose weight, analyze a brand new skill, or quite smoking, consuming, or taking tablets. The satisfactory way to introduce alternate for your lifestyles is to take it one small step at a time.

As a final note on this chapter, bear in mind that the ultimate thing you want to do is to overexert your already tired eyes. If you sense that you are straining too much, then drop your training activities and palm your eyes. You should comply with through with a fab towel for properly measure.

Don't strain your self an excessive amount of with the sports. Learn to take it smooth and loosen up.

NVI GOOD EYE HABITS

So now you recognize the fundamental eye-rest and eye-strengthening sports in our Natural Vision Improvement application, as well as the basic outline of what you need to do on a every day basis.

But these types of sporting activities could be for naught if you don't recognise a way to take suitable care of your eyes within the first region.

Natural Vision Improvement isn't about just doing a couple of minutes of scheduled physical games and spending the relaxation of the day doing matters that harm your eyes.

It's approximately mastering a new manner to apply your eyes, if you want to maintain them in incredible shape for the rest of your life.

The eye physical games already noted in this e-book will automatically train your eyes to feature extra efficaciously in the course of the day, but there are sure things that could't be described as sports, but alternatively, as habits which you adopt through the years and use all through the day.

By cultivating appropriate eye conduct, you make sure that you maintain and even improve your eyesight robotically as time is going through. So ensure you keep the following guidelines in mind:

Get More Sunshine In Your Life

If you've been analyzing this guide cautiously, you may word that I recommended you get at the least to three hours of outdoor light. Even if you don't bask inside the solar, simply staying exterior will get some top old style daylight bouncing into your eyes.

This is important for maintaining your eyes healthful as our eyes have advanced to better adapt to herbal daylight. Depriving your eyes of daylight will ultimately cause them to warp out of shape – which is why bookworms, office-people, net junkies and video-game addicts have a tendency to broaden a whole range of eye problems, and why you so regularly see them carrying glasses (although nowadays, in case you appearance greater intently, you'll notice even more of them sporting touch lenses).

Artificial light from bulbs, TV's, laptop screens, phones and different devices, simply can not reflect the herbal light of the solar in conjunction with its herbal benefits in your eyes.

And except, the greater vitamin D gained from sunlight in conjunction with the bodily exercise (of each your frame and eyes) you get whilst staying outside will do you a world of desirable.

At Least Get As Much Light As Possible

Okay, so no longer anyone has the luxury of spending two to 3 hours in the extremely good outside. Also, a whole lot of oldsters are caught having to stare at a laptop display all day, because it's a part of their job.

If you need to work indoors for prolonged durations of time, then the least you can do is to provide enough mild so that you don't ought to squint and pressure your eyes. Make sure this mild isn't without delay aimed toward your eyes even though, as this could stress your eyes even greater.

This is a specially critical idea to don't forget in case you stay in the front of a TV or computer screen for prolonged periods of time. This light can 'burn' the fovea centralis as well as region tremendous quantities of pressure on the ciliary muscles. It is because of this that you have to use a brilliant enough room light to counter the light emitted by way of the screen.

Oh, and don't overlook the 10-twenty rule whilst operating. It'll do wonders on your eyes ultimately.

Get Enough Sleep

A no-brainer on the subject of appropriate eye conduct is getting sufficient sleep. This is the time while all of the elements of your body – specifically the eyes – are, for the most element, shut down and given time to get over the day's stressors.

Good sleep is essential on your health and for your eyes.

Some parents say that five or six hours of sleep are sufficient, whilst others insist that you surely want eight hours of sleep. The high-quality rule of thumb here is to get sufficient sleep so you awaken feeling fine and fresh. This is due to the fact some human beings, such as the elderly, definitely can't sleep extra than six hours, whilst others need to nod off for 8 to nine hours in order to awaken feeling notable.

That first rate feeling is what you want when you wake up, so be aware of what number of hours you slept every time you wake up with that excellent feeling.

Be ware of slumbering too lengthy though, as research display this can damage your fitness by way of increasing your threat of heart sickness and different illnesses.

Eat Right

You are what you eat – and what you consume influences your eyesight.

Food received't offer a short-restoration to your eye troubles, however an eye fixed-pleasant eating regimen will provide your eyes the vitamins they need to stay in top notch shape.

So what ingredients should you devour on your eyes?

Anything that includes the following additives: nutrition C, diet A, vitamin E, folic acid, zinc and selenium. Most of those can be found in not unusual vegetables, so ensure you add masses of carrots, broccoli, bell peppers, Brussels sprouts and spinach for your food plan.

One fantastic-food that I've currently been experimenting with and had incredible effects with my clients and with my personal eyes, is the Indian spice, turmeric.

Turmeric is especially top at boosting your imaginative and prescient, because it has more than one effective actions on your eyes. It is a effective anti-oxidant, a effective anti inflammatory, a effective anti-estrogen, and it additionally thins your blood, thereby growing the blood-glide for your eyes.

You can upload turmeric in your food, but it's a whole lot of trouble, and I've found the first-class manner to take it is in supplement shape. Below is the complement that I'm presently the usage of and it's the first-class one I've tried thus far for my eyes (I've tried dozens):

If you don't live in both the U.S. Or the U.K. Simply attempt any other turmeric with bioperine or black pepper extract. You would possibly should attempt some exclusive ones until you discover one which works well with enhancing your eyesight.

On the meatier facet of things, make sure that you get greater turkey, sardines and wild salmon into your weight-reduction plan. You can also add some sweet potatoes on your weight loss plan. Bake a few of these and you can either snack on them or upload them to your important food for the day.

A exact preferred rule of thumb with regards to weight loss plan and improving your eyesight, is to eat more non-starchy greens!

Oh, and recollect to cut down on the ingredients that do greater harm than top for your frame. Foods wealthy in sugar, caffeine, alcohol and occasional-density lipid (LDL) cholesterol not only do damage to the diverse organs of your body, but they also make it tougher on your body to higher take in the aforementioned vitamins as properly.

Practice Not Depending On Visual Aids

Glasses and get in touch with lenses have their uses. You will nonetheless depend on them until your eyesight gets higher, particularly whilst you want to be in top shape for tasks like using or working. You do, but, need to recognise that visible aids are supposed to be a crutch – no longer an answer – on your vision issues.

It is for this reason which you want to discover ways to characteristic and move around with out relying too heavily on your visual aids. It will take a few getting used to and also you won't be able to do the whole thing proper off the bat, however that is the handiest actual way you will be able to regain your eyesight.

If you don't practice getting round without visual aids, then your state of affairs is similar to a bedridden affected person – the muscle mass will in the end atrophy to the point in which they emerge as too susceptible to characteristic properly.

A Note On Vision Therapy

There is every other approach of improving your eyesight known as vision therapy, additionally referred to as imaginative and prescient education. It is a miles greater advanced version of the Natural Vision Improvement software, but you will need the offerings of a mainly-educated optometrist to conduct vision therapy.

Both applications are similar in the sort of way that they use sporting activities to help you see higher. The primary distinction is that imaginative and prescient therapy also desires quite a few specialized gadget – filters, lenses, prisms, occluders and pc packages – to keep tune of your progress. I notably recommend which you are seeking the offerings of an optometrist who makes a speciality of vision remedy.

I'm now not announcing that imaginative and prescient remedy is superior or that NVI is much less effective. The close steerage of a expert is always an excellent aspect, particularly considering NVI and imaginative and prescient therapy percentage the same fundamental roots. A skilled specialist can better manual you along the bits and bobs of eye sports.

It's simply which you first want to locate an optometrist specializing in vision therapy. Once you do, then you need as a way to have the funds for his/her services for numerous months. That's a major trouble of imaginative and prescient therapy – one which doesn't exist with NVI.

Chapter 5: Structure Of The Eye

The human eye has a comparable layout to a projector. There is a lens within the the front, and there's a display on the back. A projector lens is truely a sequence of lenses, that make sure that the image shows up without a doubt behind the display. The eye lens is connected to a muscle, that elongates or relaxes the eye. This causes the focal duration of the lens to trade. This guarantees that a sharp picture suggests up at the retina. Also there are a sequence of lenses round the attention, that purpose the eye to elongate or loosen up. This again has the impact of adjusting the focal duration of the attention.

The human eye is a awesome piece of engineering. It is designed to be used in many numerous lighting environments. For this dialogue, I'll generalize a bit. The eye is designed to work in five distinctive ways. Low mild, vivid light, near imaginative and prescient, a ways vision, and peripheral vision.

There are sorts of receptors in the attention. One for low light and one for bright mild. The light levels correspond to full moon and brilliant sunlight. The human eye has been designed to modify between these extremes, robotically. A digicam can file light stages of 6 f stops. The human eye can do 12.

The eye can also also consciousness on some distance gadgets and near objects. The muscle groups in the eye modify the focal duration of the eye via stretching. In a herbal relaxed state, the eye lens can see gadgets over 20 toes away, with out being stretched. In technical terms, this would be taken into consideration infinity for the attention.

In the middle of the eye there may be a area called the macula. This region has a excessive concentration of sensors and nerves. So this region is used to make out details.

Most of what we name seeing occurs within the mind. The mind integrates the pics from both eyes into stereo vision. The eye scans photographs around twenty instances a 2nd. The mind fuses these pix to create one non-stop picture. The thoughts additionally adjusts for lighting fixtures, and decides which sensor stay on or off. It decodes the information and makes experience of the photos. It adjusts the eye muscle groups in order that the picture is sharp at the retina.

It is a fallacy to accept as true with the thoughts is localized inside the head. The complete human body is sensible. Every cell in body has a sure intelligence constructed into it. This is just like way present day gadget consisting of cars are designed. Modern automobiles have gadgets which includes tire pressure sensor, multiple microprocessors, audio structures and pretty frequently a significant microprocessor. It might be wrong to assume that every one the processing takes place within the central processor. The thoughts of the human is spread in the complete frame.

The seeing element is likewise depends on different human beings close by. One may finish that what we see depends on different humans.

On a trekking ride lately, one of the guys pointed to item and stated that a certain historic residence become located there. All people agreed that we ought to see it. Back domestic, I tried to do a web look for it, however turned into unable to discover it. I trust all us were a part of the identical wondering system and as a result noticed some thing that didn't exist.

When the ciliary muscle mass that preserve the lens relaxes, the lens is flat and lets in for remote imaginative and prescient. When the object you're looking at is closer than twenty feet away, those muscle tissues contract the lens assumes a spherical shape. This is called accommodation.

Irregularly shaped eyeballs are the motive of the 2 maximum not unusual vision issues, myopia and hyperopia.

The eye can be as compared to a camera and its element. It is approximately round and packed with fluids. The eye while developed is prepared for consciousness at infinity. An eye longer than common is nearsighted or myopic. This can cognizance objects carefully but receives blurry while focuses a long way. An eye this is shorter than average is farsighted or hyperopic. This eye can attention some distance honestly, but not close to.

The eye focal lengths are measured in diopters. An eye with 2 diopters can awareness at ½ meter. A myopic eye can recognition earlier than this period. A hyperopic eye can recognition past this distance.

So how does the eye exchange its cognizance? The very the front of the eye is the cornea. Behind the cornea is the scholar forming iris tissue. Behind the student is the eye lens. How the attention focuses, is a supply of controversy. Some authors claim it's due to the eye lens converting shape. Some declare it's due to the muscle tissues of the attention stretching or relaxing the eye.

The cornea is the clear rounded the front part of the eye. Since it's far obvious, it can not be seen with the bare eye, until regarded from the aspect. The cornea has no blood vessels, however receives nutrition from tears and the aqueous fluid bathing its inner floor. When wholesome it is as clean as glass. Being rounded, it plays a element in focusing the mild. However unlike the lens, the cornea cannot exchange form to consciousness the eye.

If the cornea is greater elongated like a soccer, the eye has astigmatism. This is pretty regular. Minor quantities of astigmatism might not require the use of glasses.

When mild strikes the cornea, it's miles transmitted thru the scholar. The student features like an aperture in a camera, which turns into large or smaller to let in special amounts of light. The pupil is the colored part of the attention. The pupil serves to shield the interior of the eye from overexposure.

The iris has a dense black pigmented layer at the out of doors. This is the same for all and sundry. There is not any such thing as blue, green or hazel eyes. The the front layer is irregular and can from pure white to brown. While imposed onto black gives the arrival of blue eyes. Different amounts of pigments cause the attention to appear to have distinct hues.

The colour of the attention modifications depending on the dimensions of the student. In vibrant mild the pupil is mall and what

97

pigment is on the the front floor is rather scattered, making the eye colour lighter. When large the scholar size reasons the pigment to compress, causing the attention to color darker.

Behind the lens is a huge cavity full of vitreous fluid. This is a thick clean gel, made up of broadly speaking water. It is apparent and optically transmits mild thru the pupil and lens.

The retina is a skinny layer or nerve tissue lining the internal of the back two thirds of the attention. It is corresponding to a film in a digital camera. It is made of cells referred to as rods and cones. The small center inside the lower back of the eye is called the macula. It is where the light is focused. It consists of simplest cones. In the periphery of the retina, it's far completed fabricated from rods. The rods are vital for night imaginative and prescient, movement and peripheral imaginative and prescient.

The optic nerve enters the back of the attention in the direction of the nostril from the macula. The mind techniques the pictures, from the eye. It reverses upside down photos, and creates stereoscopic vision. The left mind sees matters to the right and proper mind sees matters to the left.

So what is everyday vision? 20/20 vision is considered as the standard. It means that at 20 toes, you should be capable of see at 20 feet. Similarly, 20/40 imaginative and prescient manner that at 20 toes, you should see at 40 toes. This is the minimum to accumulate a riding license in most states. Legal blindness method 20/2 hundred even with glasses, at any distance. There is any such element as supernormal imaginative and prescient. Its imaginative and prescient higher than 20/20 vision.

It's an oversimplification to evaluate the attention to a digital camera, but it gives an affordable starting point. When you direct the attention to an object, it captures an photograph of the retina. The lens enables to attention the image on the retina.

In creation, the eye Is a 3 layered ball. The inner layer is the retina. The center layer is the choroid, that's a maze of blood vessels that feed the eye. The outermost layer is a difficult protective tissue known as sclera, and is popularly call the white of the attention. It's opaque besides for a obvious place in the the front called the cornea.

When the light is going past the cornea, it arrives at the iris. This is a flexible diaphragm with a transparent center, the student. As it expands or contracts the pupil, the iris controls the amount of light entering farther into the attention.

After the iris, the mild rays pass via the lens which refracts or bends them, so that focus on the middle of the attention. The rays arrive at the retina after a going thru the vitreous body.

The retina incorporates forty five million receptors known as cones and rods. The cones are heavily concentrated in a small place known as the macula, and maximum of that is within the fovea. The rods are involved with the night time seeing, and they placed faraway from the macula.

As the rods and cones receive mild, every receptor selections up a fraction of the image and transmits it to the brain. The mind combines those right into a unmarried photo. This is some distance greater complex than whatever human beings have invented.

In the most commonplace form of faulty imaginative and prescient, mild rays aren't targeted sharply on the retina, and a blur results. When the rays are delivered to their sharpest attention, in the front of the retina, close to sightedness results. When the rays are focused so that they're focused at the back of the retina, a ways sightedness consequences.

There are numerous theories on how the rays are centered. One concept is that, the ciliary muscle groups around the eye, adjust the lens, in order that the eye focuses effectively. Another concept is that the muscle tissues around the eye contract or amplify the eye ball, to obtain attention. The 2d concept is credited to William Bates. He said that on account that the attention muscle groups are controlled via nerve impulses, he said that reducing strain and learning to peer, can restoration imaginative and prescient problems.

CAUSES OF EYE PROBLEMS

Earlier, I had stated how handiest the geeks in my magnificence, wore glasses. I'm certain a lot of you, assumed that handiest exact college students wore glasses. It's authentic! The eye is designed to appearance some distance. The eye muscular tissues loosen up and might without problems look far. Looking near all the time reasons the attention to alter itself to look near. This reasons degeneration of the ability to cognizance a ways. My determine's technology by no means spent that tons time in front of the TV, reading, on a pc or playing video video games. This reasons them to appearance a long way.

Once upon a time, the human eye become perfectly designed to serve the needs of humans. People could hunt, farm, or sew clothes, without optical crutches. People by and large communicated thru speech. Those had been the times that royalty have been now not required to be literate. Then people learned to communicate through analyzing, and everyone become required to wait school. Everyone was predicted to examine and write. There are books and writing everywhere. Some well printed, a few published badly. Suddenly every body became forced to put on glasses

When youngsters start school, they may be all of sudden thrown right into a lecture room scenario, in which adjustment to a new way of dwelling, causes lines and terrible seeing conduct. As we grow old, similarly stress and tension give a boost to horrific seeing behavior.

Clara Hackett ran a survey of a hundred hundred excessive college students. The questions had been approximately when they noticed eye loss, and what came about at that time. Eighty percent said that that they had misplaced eye sight due to an emotional crisis.

One of the alternative issues of sporting glasses is that it the eye stays very desk bound. This reasons a lack of sparkle in the eye. This as defined earlier is because the glasses recognition handiest on a very slim region. So the eye adjusts by means of preserving eye searching instantly beforehand. This also has a facet effect of decreasing peripheral vision. Although I can see extra actually directly beforehand, I'm now ignoring the occasions on the outer edge.

I locate that if I take my glasses off and stay existence without it, the sparkle returns very quickly. My peripheral vision improves. This has the effect of enhancing imaginative and prescient.

Remember, the antique advice on now not studying within the darkish? It's real. The eye is not designed to study in the darkish. What maximum folks try to do is examine in the night time, with the mild turned on. I discover that in vivid daylight, I can study a e-book, pretty clearly at everyday reading distance. However beneath artificial mild, I want to brilliant the e book plenty nearer or wear a set of glasses. I believe the eye is designed to be used for searching close simplest below herbal sunlight.

Until synthetic lighting came along, humans did all their seeing and activities in shiny daylight. And at night, they used moon mild or candle light to find their way round. Everyone was an afternoon man or woman. Nowadays all of us is expected to a day and night time creature. Work all day and birthday celebration all night time. The eye does now not get any rest! The shiny mild sensors in the eye get used all day. The low mild sensors never get utilized in moon light. The eye glasses make certain that we additionally best use the middle of the attention. The periphery is in no way used.

The artificial light in workplaces and homes, comes someplace among sunlight and moonlight. Using this light, as soon as a small range of the vision of the eye is used. This causes good sized fatigue in the eye, and contributes partially to imaginative and prescient problems. I actually have determined that stepping searching faraway from the computer each 15 minutes and stepping out of the workplace into sunlight every ninety mins reduces strain on the eye significantly.

In the beyond I actually have used transition lenses that darken in bright daylight. These lenses take over the function of the eye to alter. It took my eyes almost three years to discover ways to adjust once more. Use of solar shades for the eyes is almost equally bad. This prevents the eye, from running naturally in vivid daylight. The most effective time I have determined use for sunglasses is while exterior in wilderness sand or snow. I locate the light too brilliant for my eyes.

The eye turned into by no means designed to paintings below these situations. Because of synthetic lights we have night time existence. We work overdue hours. The eye in no way rests. When became the final time we learnt to loosen up by means of looking the moon?

The eye is designed to work most of the time, whilst specializing in some distance gadgets. However in our modern world, we spent a lot time studying and searching at a laptop. Or looking TV. The eye isn't always given sufficient relaxation, to loosen up and unstretch the lens. So the eye adapts in order that it now sees near objects absolutely, however not some distance items. If the variation isn't always symmetric, we get astigmatism. This means that we have extraordinary pix on two special axes. This causes double imaginative and prescient.

Unfortunately in present day life-style, the crucial location or macula is used a lot. Eye glasses provide you with clear imaginative and prescient whilst looking instantly in advance, so that the photograph is centered at the center of the attention. What occurs is that the rest of the attention is not used. This effects within the geek look, that each person who put on glasses too long should address. What this reasons is undue pressure on the eyes.

Another less regarded truth is that the glass or lenses take in some the mild. So mild visible via the lenses is much less excessive than without. Also because of adjustments in refraction of the glasses, a number of the even as mild will get cut up. So it is at times advisable to peer with out glasses to verify the original thought.

It is likewise widely recognized that human eyes dislike glasses. We usually get instructed we need to get used to them. It normally takes me two weeks to get cushty in a new pair of glasses. My eyes never commonplace contacts. After two attempts, I in no way attempted again. I pay attention that the contemporary contacts have suppressants to save you the attention from rejecting them.

All glasses reduce the sector of imaginative and prescient. Modern lenses are a lot better than the ones I used to wear. But nevertheless, my field of imaginative and prescient is a lot better with out glasses that I can placed up with the blurry vision. One of the facet effects is that we appearance instantly on and get the "geek stare". This prevents a huge part of the attention from being used.

It is constantly assumed that we need 20/20 imaginative and prescient, to live well. To qualify for a license in California, one desires handiest 20/40 vision. When we go to the attention medical doctor, he gives us a prescription that corrects for 20/20. Here's the capture. The take a look at is performed in a dark room, that simulates night time situations. As I said earlier than, we are not designed for clean night imaginative and prescient. Although we'd have 20/20 imaginative and prescient in large sunlight hours, within the testing room, our vision dims to 20/40. So we get a brand new set of glasses. And we get instructed that we want it all of the time, in any other case our imaginative and prescient will go to pot. So in the day time we now adjust to the brand new glasses. So what was now best 20/20 in vast daylight is now a 20/40 or worse vision. And now night time vision deteriorates correspondingly. Hence it's a by no means ending cycle of new lenses.

I don't forget going to my eye health practitioner to get a 20/forty correction. I referred to I wished that because I become seeking to enhance my imaginative and prescient. She located it funny. She become MD, and advised me that studies had disproved any vision development packages. She had attempted it but nothing happened. I were given the lenses anyway.

The biggest cause of vision loss is day by day stress. As mentioned before, most of the seeing occurs in the mind. Our mind fuses the two pix into one. It adjusts the eye lenses to get a clean vision. So when the computer in us, miscalculates, we get blurry imaginative and prescient. Stress comes in all bureaucracy. At work, at domestic, while riding, searching at a pc and nearly everything cutting-edge people do. Blurry imaginative and prescient for a while is ordinary. It takes place to anybody. We don't want new glasses then. Instead we need to get rid of the supply of the strain. Once removed, imaginative and prescient improves.

As stated, the complete body is clever. Stress on the frame, disorder, or flawed meals causes more strain at the frame. This in turn will purpose blurry vision. I find that every time I fall unwell or have a carrying injury or paintings an excessive amount of time beyond regulation, my vision turns blurry. I study in a newspaper of a few character, whose imaginative and prescient advanced drastically, after his lower back ache were given dealt with.

Its not unusual expertise that multiplied TV, computers and video games reasons vision to get blurry. In addition to the whole thing I have said, the photos on the TV aren't consistent images like we see in the bodily global. The snap shots are suspended in air. Our eye and mind cannot surely decide wherein the photo exactly is. Also the photograph receives refreshed more than one times a 2nd. This flicker causes the thoughts to now not method photos successfully. Over prolonged durations, this could eye stress, headaches and thicker glasses.

We get clear imaginative and prescient handiest while the stresses on the attention, mind and frame are eliminated.

There are lots of facts to expose that nearly everybody suffer from defective vision after the age of 20. When as soon as, primitive guy had suitable eyesight, we suffer from horrific vision at a younger age. Use of eyeglasses and different optical crutches do no longer gradual the imaginative and prescient troubles.

When the eye looks at familiar objects it is comfortable and below no stress. However while we see an surprising, the attention is below greater strain and this causes brief eye defects. Unfamiliar scripts, or maps would additionally cause pressure. Changes in light intensity, or publicity to sturdy mild will motive imperfect sight. Imagine entering into vibrant daylight from a dark room or vice versa.

Interestingly loud noise or changes in background noise cause modifications in vision. Mental or bodily soreness, sickness, modifications in temperature.

I usually discover it tough maintaining the glasses clean. Rain, perspiration and water condensation can cloud the lenses. And there are the scratches from touch. These result in eye stress and complications.

Imperfect vision is because of pressure in the attention. Glasses do now not relieve the pressure in the eye. They best make it worse or make the stress permanent. Sometimes I assume that glasses are more like mental guidelines as opposed to actual therapies.

The eye can see in reality most effective inside the valuable location, the macula. Under strain, the center of the eye blanks out. Under extreme conditions the man or woman can see the identical from the middle of the eye, and the edges of the attention. This is called eccentric fixation. This can reason outstanding pressure on the attention. Normal vision is one in all crucial fixation. Under principal fixation, the eyes and thoughts are relaxed. And no dark circles form underneath the eyes. Under intense pressure, nervous fluttering of the eyelids and redness of the attention may also occur

We are not born with 20/20 vision. As infants broaden, they get higher vision. Eventually they get stereo imaginative and prescient and colour vision.

There are many eye diseases that can't be solved the use of the techniques described. Below are a number of the common ones.

The detection of amblyopia or lazy eye is one of the principal motives for vision screening in younger youngsters. The amblyopic eye is structurally normal but does now not see properly inspite of glasses. This is also referred to as go eyes.

There are many causes of crimson eye. A not unusual contamination is referred to as conjunctivitis. This influences the outer vascular layer of tissue masking the attention. This is pretty commonplace among school kids. The regular symptom is a purple eye.

When the attention is much redder, it is probably a symptom of spontaneous conjuctival hemorrhage. The redness may additionally seem pretty extreme. However the redness is localized typically to one part of the attention. The man or woman wakes up and looks within the replicate. It normally does now not have any fitness importance. The biggest trouble is to guarantee human beings that there is no problem. Episleritis and Iritis are typically quite similar.

Scleritis and acute glaucoma is a deeper layer irritation than the above. It is the infection of the white of the eye itself. The redness is localized, but the pain is extreme. Medical care is required.

Foreign body sensations, take place whilst items can enter the attention, that allows you to stick with the attention. This may be not unusual to people using drilling or slicing tools. It's possible to take away the foreign our bodies via washing the eye, or batting the attention lids. It's additionally feasible to have these sensations with touch lenses.

There are pretty a few viruses and bacteria that motive eye infection. An example being the herpes easy virus

Dry eye is a totally not unusual problem. Tears are herbal lubricants, fashioned through the conjuctival glands and the lacrimal glands. Tear production is fairly regular from conjuctival glands, but can be suffering from sicknesses of the conjunctiva. Dry eye is usually resulting from tear manufacturing via the conjunctival glands. It is also a symptom of Lasik surgical procedure.

Spots inside the vision, which move with the motion of the eye, in a floating manner, are referred to as floaters. They constitute a minor nuisance. They are pretty not unusual whilst visible in opposition to a mild colored wall. However a large onset of floaters would imply a scientific condition. It can be retinal detachment or something else that calls for medical treatment.

A spot inside the vision that seems desk bound may be some thing more widespread. This is probably due to a swelling of the macula, or other degeneration. If growth happens on the cornea, those want to be surgically eliminated.

Strabismus or move eyed can be genetic or from damage. The most common age related problem is cataract. Cataracts are modern blockading out of the eye. This is usually surgically eliminated.

Another commonplace age related eye ailment is glaucoma. Glaucoma occurs due to the fact the intraocular pressure builds. A visual view trying out peripheral vision, with computerized strategies, can discover glaucoma.

Macular degeneration affects 2 to three percent of the populace. As you can don't forget, the macula is the relevant part of the attention. This degeneration is valuable. It generally affects reading and shade vision. Since the peripheral vision is undamaged, it means, that sometime humans see from the facet of the eye. Such human beings can't look you in the attention.

Vascular occlusion is because of the arteries or veins to the eye, suddenly constricting. This causes excessive imaginative and prescient losses, additionally known as a stroke of the eye. Sometimes this is probably because of high cholesterol buildup.

Swelling of the optic nerve can occur due to numerous motives. It can be from beginning, tumors or injuries. Other not unusual neurological issues encompass multiple sclerosis, double imaginative and prescient, and complications.

It is generally assumed that refractive residences of the eye never change. At the flip of the nineteenth century, a ophthalmologist named William Bates, conducted a chain of studies at the motives for the errors of refraction. He used an device referred to as the retinoscope, to without a doubt look at the adjustments within the refraction of the attention. Most of his studies was largely forgotten through the years, in reality as it contradicted mainstream thoughts and threatened the attention glass enterprise.

According to his research, refractive index of the eye modifications for the duration of the day. The numerous defects of the eye, namely long sight, short sight and astigmatism might be seem and disappear at some stage in the day. His research showed him that these had been produced because of improper movement of the muscular tissues around the eye. His research also confirmed that in spite of ideal sight, the residences of the eye changed at some stage in the day. That is one ought to have short sight and long sight at some stage in a single day. Research on infants shows similar consequences.

Errors of refraction will increase all through sleep. So humans with normal imaginative and prescient will faulty vision during sleep. So it's possible to wake up within the morning with eyes extra worn-out that before sleep. Research additionally indicates that after person is unconscious because of Ether, chloroform, refractive errors nevertheless show up.

To me, which means I have clean vision in the course of the morning. As I get greater tired my imaginative and prescient blurs. With some rest, my vision receives clearer. My eye also receives full-size relaxation, after I take my glasses off.

No eye specialist or eye health practitioner can declare that eye glasses are greater than a crutch. They offer symptom relief, however do now not touch the reasons of defects.

Eyeglasses are inconvenient, and produce adjustments in seems. They impose restraints on sports. They are annoying once they fog. They should get replaced, while broken. If you've got faulty vision and worn glasses for a long time, then it's in all likelihood that, you've got used several prescriptions, and each time stronger. The not unusual even though is that vision deteriorates and gets worse with age. Hence want for stronger prescriptions. There are many like me, that eyeglasses make the hassle worse. Maybe that explains why they fail for two thirds of the populace.

In the "higher vision now", Clara Hackett, indicates creating a card, with pinholes separated by way of three/sixteen inch apart.

Now hold the auto before your eyes, and look through the pinholes. Try looking casually. I could in reality see certainly!

I had more capacity imaginative and prescient than I found out. This exercises illustrates which you had to centralize you imaginative and prescient, and make your eyes extra mobile. It has been lengthy held that the mistakes are because of defects in the lens or because of defects within the muscles that maintain the attention and lenses. I believe that to many like me defective imaginative and prescient isn't due to a fault in the eye however because of flawed use of the eyes.

If you have got completed the pinhole test, this represents what your immediate capability sight. This is the sight unaided by pinholes or glasses. This is the development that is viable for both myopia and hyperopia.

It has lengthy been familiar principle that once refractive mistakes are because of a defective lens, or other abnormalities of the eye. The solution has been to accurate for those errors with glasses. The pinhole exams offers wish that the mistake can be greater due to gaining knowledge of the way to see efficaciously in place of structural defects in the eye. Clara Hackett says that use of vision improvement sporting activities has helped her sufferers double the vision. So someone with 20/forty can now see 20/20 imaginative and prescient. She mentions out of 2857 college students, full-size majority had improved their visions appreciably. Some may want to even pass the skip the driver's check without glasses. She also mentions that people with glaucoma and cataracts have proven splendid improvements in their imaginative and prescient. These sporting activities are not supposed to cure growths or sicknesses. It is necessary to are searching for hospital therapy.

The vision improvement physical activities are not long complex physical games. They are designed to enhance vision naturally, by using relaxation. These physical activities are a primary step and can be practiced ordinary, in the whole thing we do. You will finally learn how to discard glasses. Initially it's feasible to go brief durations without glasses, and subsequently extend the time with out it. The development in vision happens depends at the motivation to pursue vision improvement.

There are some more dividends. Near sighted humans frequently tend to be shy, and tackle new stature as their vision improves. Many farsighted people appear to be problem of high-quality apprehensive anxiety that reasons them to transport too rapidly. As their sight improves they're mentally and physically calmer.

On a screen the size of a teaspoon bowl, a ordinary eye can see miles of landscape, or study great print in a ebook. Seeing is a intellectual in addition to a bodily skill. It is a talent received by way of us. New born infants are born nearly blind, and learn to see.

HOW TO IMPROVE VISION

From the previous segment, it have to be obvious that the motives for blurry vision are many. All can trace returned to unsuitable use of the eyes, mind and body. So to get clean vision, one has to dispose of all of the external stresses. Several research have proven that one's vision does blurrier with age, due to increasing stress. Studies have also shown that use of eye glass will increase, as literacy, computer systems and TV boom in recognition.

I'm completely for literacy. Otherwise I won't be writing this. I examine voraciously. I watch TV once in a while. I paintings on a laptop. My imaginative and prescient maintains enhancing.

The largest stress at the eyes is the eye glasses. I discover that if I wear glasses for extra than 50 minutes, my eyes start hurting. From the previous sections, glasses reason one to have a fixed stare and reason the "geek" look.

I find that to lessen the strain, I take my glasses off for 10 minutes each hour and cover my eyes. I then visualize perfect blackness. Black as a night sky with no stars. I think imagine stars coming on one by one. After 10 mins, I find that my eyes have comfortable. Another aspect I do is to region the glasses on decrease down on my nose, in order that it now capabilities as studying glasses.

I additionally trained myself to do as plenty as feasible with out glasses. I started out out by using trying to walk around my house. It took me months to do this without bumping into things and those. I also attempted consuming without making a mess. That took time. I then graduated onto other sports, house paintings, walks round my rental complex and even seeking to examine a e-book. I find that it's a great deal easier a book in vibrant sunlight than in the shade or with synthetic lighting. I can currently maintain a ebook at arm's period and study in sunlight. I want to maintain the e book within 6 inches in artificial light.

The largest venture become learning to go a street again. Initially I had a difficult time judging the rate of motors, and seeing the site visitors lights to pass the street. This took some time. I tried to parent out as a whole lot as feasible. I kept the glasses in my hand and verified yes, that I had seen correctly. I took me nearly six months to cross a chief intersection with out glasses or with out someone else.

Once I had self belief to pass a avenue, I tried to do greater. I love to hike outside. I did a ten mile alone in one in all my preferred parks without glasses. I took a few months to accumulate the self belief. I had a trouble analyzing the signs and symptoms from a distance. Nothing says that I cannot read path signs and symptoms from 3 toes away.

I decided to get extra adventurous. I changed into going to motorbike to work, with out glasses. This became taking large risks. I knew the route, site visitors was low and there have been motorcycle lanes. I had come this a ways, why not take one extra step.

I don't forget getting on my motorcycle and wondering "Arun, You labored this hard and have a vehicle, and a super set of glasses. Just pressure". I started out cycling. It changed into super. I hadn't biked to paintings when you consider that university. I nevertheless do that regularly.

I take into account getting up the next day and wondering that I need to attempt to play football once more. This became harder. I couldn't spot the ball or the goals too nicely. The players paintings either white shirts or black shirts. So I could inform my group. I soon realized that even though I had fuzzy imaginative and prescient, I had lots higher peripheral imaginative and prescient. And my eyes were extra relaxed. No extra broken frames.

I asked my tennis companion, if she didn't mind hitting with me. Since I turned into extra skilled, this grew to become out to be a good game.

This was terrific. I ought to now play recreation with out glasses. Finally!

The one component I could now not ever do is driving with out glasses. It's a recipe for catastrophe. I always use the prescribed lenses while using.

My lens energy went from 4.25(left)/four.50(proper) to a few.Five(left).3.Seventy five(right). Astigmatism stayed the equal. I hit a plateau. I was now existence quite a big part of my existence without glasses. I nevertheless had blurry imaginative and prescient.

Exercise:

If you've been the use of glasses for a long time, this can be hard. Everyday attempt taking your glasses off for 10 minutes. Allow yourself to relax.

When you get used to this, attempt on foot throughout your condominium. This can take a few being used to. It made me a better housekeeper, in preparation for this exercise

Slowly attempt increasing the number of activities which you do without glasses. This will take time and persistence.

I commenced dwelling more healthy. I started out cooking. More spices, vegetables, and much less meat. I ate out less. I did yoga physical activities frequently. My body aches and stiffness disappeared. I found out that it is crucial to exercise and stretch all of the muscle tissue in my body. This is quite exceptional from Northern California, wherein humans think in terms of marathons and hard bodies. Muscles are predicted to be soft. That will increase range of motion. Human beings are designed for a wide range of motion. Being buff and rock hard decreases the variety of movement. I've also study that having over advanced outer muscular tissues beneath develops the internal muscle groups. The human frame is designed as an natural whole. Everything is interconnected. Everything has a purpose and use.

Exercise:

Another set of sporting activities, that I located beneficial are sporting events for the attention. Move your eye, so that pupil is now at the pinnacle, searching upward. Now rotate the eye, so that the pupil is rotating one loop clockwise across the periphery. Now rotate the eye counterclockwise once. Repeat the workout 10 times.

Exercise:

Now pass the attention to the right fringe of the eye. Move it quickly to the left side. And to the right. Repeat 10 times.

Now flow the attention to the top. Move quickly to the bottom. And to the pinnacle. Now repeat 10 instances.

Exercise:

Focus on a close to item, around five cm from the eye. Focus on an item some distance away, like a distant constructing. And now consciousness on a close to object. Repeat 10 instances.

Exercise:

In brilliant daylight near your eyes, and flow your face, so that you're dealing with the solar. The eyes stay shut constantly. Move your face backward and forward, in order that the sun is going over every eye. Do this 10 instances. Now pass interior to a darker room.

This will help the eye to modify over unique light degrees.

I determined to improve my night vision. I turned down the lighting fixtures in my apartment, and installed night time lights in my apartments. I opened the windows to permit in moonlight. I even attempted moon light hikes with out a glasses and no flashlights. I controlled to hike one of the neighborhood peaks under moonlight. It became excellent!

Exercise

This exercise is to improve my low mild imaginative and prescient. At night time flip down the lighting, and until you have moonlight for your room. If that doesn't paintings, attempt the use of night time lamps. Now wait till your eyes regulate. Look on the the items in the room and notice what number of you could pick out. Once you're comfortable doing that, try walking throughout the room

Although my peripheral imaginative and prescient became now enhancing, I found out that there was more that might be carried out. I tried taping a black cardboard simply above my eyebrow, in order that it blocked my critical vision.

Exercise

Here's an exercising to improve peripheral vision. Tape a piece of black cardboard to so that it covers the middle of each your eyes. So now you could handiest see using your peripheral vision. Try doing a little of your each day sports this manner. Start with ten minutes and boom the time slowly.

Around this period I were given involved with japanese spirituality. I determined that I subsequently wished a few peace and quiet in my existence. I started made peace pals with own family, buddies, former employers, and former girlfriends. I pondered. I slowed my life down. I cleaned up my residence. I downsized. I slept well. I wiped clean up my life. I rearranged my office furniture in order that I ought to the whole thing changed into within easy reach. I felt more non violent. And my imaginative and prescient progressed.

As cited previously, pressure reduces the sensitivity of the center of the attention. To improve imaginative and prescient, one need to learn how to cognizance on a small area at a time. For instance, if one has to discover ways to can only see the pinnacle of a letter on this e-book certainly, and the relaxation needs to be less clear. This comes with practice. It is said that people with eagle imaginative and prescient, have a excessive diploma of important fixation. Bates mentions that crucial fixation could dispose of many eye illnesses, like glaucoma, cataract, and so on.

To be capable of see without a doubt via the center, this calls for mental manage and rest. Relaxation permits the mind to characteristic as designed.

To allow the attention to relax in the day time, considered one of easiest approaches to do this is via palming.

Exercise

Rub the fingers until it's far warm. Close the eyelids, and then vicinity the hands over the eyes. No light have to input through the fingers. Now consider the blackest nights, and believe that blackness is in the front of you. When you see perfect black, consider a vibrant famous person shining inside the center of the inky blackness. Hold this for a couple of minutes. It took me some time with a purpose to reap best blackness. And then once I did, my imaginative and prescient stepped forward hastily. In one lecture by Meir Schneider, he cited that he had patients who saw streaks of shade rather than perfect black.

When the thoughts is able to remember something perfectly, the mind and frame is relaxed. When the attention visualizes some thing properly, the eyes see perfect black, with eyes closed. Bates mentions that the quantity of black an eye sees is correlated to the quantity of imperfect vision. Usually when one sees sincerely, at a certain distance, one relaxes. However while the identical item is moved away, the person stops enjoyable and is unable to see certainly.

We see in large part with the mind, and a touch with the eyes. Everything we see is depending on the thoughts's interpretation of the photos. A man or woman looks smaller at the distance than nearby, if we don't understand him. However to a acquainted man or woman, the man or woman seems simply as large. No two people will get the identical mental photo.

When the attention is out of attention, the shape of the items may be distorted. And the shape may be distorted, depending at the day, time, strain and so forth. When the individual realizes that the photograph is an imagined one, the image may also disappear. When the individual is inclined to imagine the photo as opposed to attempt to see it, the strain disappears, and the character sees well once more. When the attention appears at a familiar item it's miles comfortable. When it looks at unusual object it traces.

Another exercising I discovered beneficial is using sunlight.

The emphasis is on casual, every day exercise, in preference to hours of drills. It's simpler training even as doing each day sports, so that it will become a part of life.

It was time to get new lenses. Same health practitioner, equal routine. I make it a point to get my imaginative and prescient examined, first element within the morning. My imaginative and prescient is continually higher in the morning. The effects are out: 2.5(left), 3.00 (proper), and astigmatism (zero/0.5).

I tried explaining what I did. This time, no smirk. I stated that the ones research she referenced didn't encompass one eccentric engineer who hated sporting glasses. And disliked surgical operation even greater so.

Relaxation can do extra than relaxation your eyes. They relieve strain and anxiety. It is the primary crucial step on the road to development. Here are some strategies that I discover useful.

Exercise in sunning

Close your eyelids and examine the sun. Move your head from one aspect to any other. This manner gets one used to bright daylight.

Having light shine on the closed lids is one of the useful of all strategies. It's beneficial all day. I decide upon sunning using direct daylight. Sunning ought to be carried out with the eyes closed.

Sit without problems to your chairs, dealing with the light, eyes closed. Turn your head gently closer to your left shoulder. From right here swing it in the direction of your proper shoulder. Keep the pinnacle perfectly poised. The total swing must cover no extra than 90 tiers. As you sun, you ought to sense a sense of relaxation, and maybe a touch drowsy.

Try to sun as frequently as you may. Have no fears approximately light. Unfortunately we're a kingdom of sunglass wearers, which can be frightened of light. If there is glare from sand or water or snow, tinted glasses may be worn. Otherwise our eyes will work perfectly properly with out them.

Sunning is helpful to the thoughts. Normally the mind is constantly concerned with the shape, colour and different aspects of items. When the eyes are closed in sunning, there may be nothing for the mind to interpret. There is simplest light. That human beings locate this so mentally restful that they end up drowsy. I'm continually amazed how clear my imaginative and prescient will become, after sunning. It was been recommended that sunning is beneficial for crossed eyes.

Exercise in Palming

The next primary aid to rest is palming. Cup the arms of each fingers over your eyes. The fingertips of one hand have to be barely crossed over those at the brow. Do now not stiffen your finds. Keep them relax. Palm even as seated easily with both ft on the floor. A pillow on your lap will help aid your elbows. If you don't have a pillow reachable, use the edges of the desk or a table. Your neck and shoulders must be relaxed.

Close your eyes when palming. Make certain your palms are unfastened and don't touch the eyes. The hands should be cupped over the eyes. Never press or rub the eyes. In this position no mild must come in. With practice it's feasible to assume blackness.

Palming helps to bring warm temperature to the eyes, and the darkness, which assist relaxation.

Exercise: The long swing.

The lengthy swing is an extremely good method to growth relaxation of the entire body. You stand straight and relaxed, without stiffness, together with your feel parallel to each other, about shoulder width apart. With your fingers placing loosely at your facets, and head degree, swing your whole frame to the left, then to the right, shifting your weight from one foot to the opposite. The entire swings should make one hundred eighty degrees. The gaze ought to comply with an imaginary horizontal eye stage line continuously, without a jumps from one object to another. You ought to get the optical illusion that the window frames are shifting in a path contrary for your swing.

Centralized vision and mobility

To get clearest vision, you need to learn to use the significant part of the attention. Learning to try this, will enhance your imaginative and prescient dramatically. The fovea is so tiny, that with ideal sight, you may see definitely only an area, the size of a dime, at normal analyzing distance. This way that nature intended vision to be a pinpointing manner involving top notch mobility. Movement is critical to imaginative and prescient. If we hold our imaginative and prescient fixated, our vision become cloudy, and we see not anything at all. Mobility and relevant fixation have to be natural and subconscious. In some cases they'll have by no means been learnt, and in some instances, they may have been misplaced.

Mobility and centralized imaginative and prescient may be regained, with exercise. Mobility and centralized imaginative and prescient typically get higher with curiosity. You could be rewarded with flashes of flawlessly clean sight. With exercise those flashes come to be everlasting.

Exercise: Counting

Counting is an terrific useful resource to expand interest and improve mobility. What may you ask must you matter? Start counting the entirety. Look around the room, and ask yourself how many gadgets are on the wall. How many gadgets are for your condo? How many coffee cups for your coworkers desk? How many stripes does each cup have?

Exercise: Edging

Edging approach searching at the rims of items to improve mobility. Edge the frames of a picture. Edge the define of leaves. As you practice edging, the hazy traces have a tendency to vanish. Practice edging the doors.

Exercise: Tossing a ball

Try tossing a ball, and follow the ball appropriately along with your eyes. You also can observe the ball in a ball sport. Try watching the ball bounce on the ground.

Exercise: Blinking

Blinking is an tremendous aid to mobility. It enables to save you staring. Blinking five to ten instances a minute is suitable.

Improving fusion

Since the eyes are 2 inches aside, every eye sees a slightly exclusive photo. The mind tries to fuse the two pics into one. Imperfect fusion is not unusual in all forms of vision loss. The improvement of fusion is an essential need to to enhancing vision.

Fusion turns into only viable, whilst the eyes transmit two photos to the mind, that lend themselves to fusion. If the attention is much less than twenty toes away, the eyes should converge upon it, turning barely turning inward. Beyond twenty feet, they must look out in parallel. If the deviation is extraordinary, and the mind doesn't suppress one photo, the end result is double vision.

Everyone's fusion goes off during quick intervals. Excessive consuming, pressure, or illness, can cause fusion to head off.

I cutting-edge civilization so much of our seeing is horizontal. Our ancestors appeared up and down, as lots as left and right. If we need to peer something to the left, we want to move our whole head to the left, in order that we will see the item with each eyes.

Here is a fusion drill that I discover beneficial.

Exercise: Cord Fusion

You will need a twenty foot duration of wire for this. Tie one end to the doorknob or to a chair at twenty toes away. Face the tied quit of the cord. Hold the cord one foot from your eyes. Now have a look at the a ways end of the twine. You need to see chords forming a V at the door knob. With a gradual downward head motion, slide your attention all of the

147

manner to the alternative end. You have to see an X fashioned through the two cords. At the end of the workout, you should see a V at your quit.

This exercising may be repeated through tying the wire vertically, and shifting your attention up and down. This exercise also can be practiced on normal gadgets. Notice the sidewalk or strength strains stretching away from you.

Facial rubdown

Ideally you ought to rub down your face by myself for at the least thirty mins. Massaging your complete face influences the circulate round your eyes.

Exercise:

Rub your arms until they're heat after which massage your face together with your fingertip, lightly at first after which more firmly. Initially the stress ought to be organization sufficient to will let you feel whether a gap is nerve-racking or painful, but to so hard that it makes it worse. Spend at the least a few minutes on every separate place, noticing how your touch feels and what effect it has.

Begin together with your jaw, and rubdown the whole region of the chin outward alongside the jawbone, in front of and at the back of the ears. You may additionally open and near the jaw whilst doing this. Massage your whole face along the cheekbones, and towards the temples, along the nostril and ears. Feel the muscle tissue loosen.

Chapter 6: Reducing Stress

As might be obvious from the previous pages, the most important source of imaginative and prescient issues is because of increasing strain. This pressure comes from multiple resources. Work, home, people, and day by day existence. These stresses may be reduced notably to reason vision improvement.

Since many of us spend a huge a part of our waking lives at work, it's miles useful to lessen pressure at paintings. For those of us who paintings at office jobs, in the front of a laptop, a few tips absolutely help. It is imperative to have a very good office chair with a couple of changes. The arm rests adjusted in order that the hands relaxation comfortably on the rests, with out soreness. Then the chair height is adjusted so that the figures are floating above the keyboard. To relaxation the arm, the fingers are placed on the wrist pad, with the palms rotated ninety stages to the keyboard.

The curvature of the backrest need to comply with the curvature of the back. The backrest have to be adjusted until this takes place.

The keyboard and mouse need to be on a keyboard tray. The monitor is adjusted in order that the consumer and may view the entire display searching slightly downward. The font length of the monitor is regularly decreased and the display back further as imaginative and prescient improves.

There are two zones of reach. The number one area which can be reached by way of shifting the arm about the elbows, and the secondary area, which requires stretching and reaching. Most the regularly used system should be inside the primary smartphone. This consists of the espresso cup, mouse, keyboard, phone, and stationary. Less frequently used equipment ought to be within the secondary zone.

It is suggested to appearance far from the display each 5 mins. It is likewise advocated to study sunlit gadgets similarly out every half-hour or so. This allows the attention to loosen up. Taking the eyeglasses out while doing this enables to relax the attention even in addition. It is helpful to stroll faraway from the table each hour or so. The human body is designed for small amounts of exchange. We don't do well doing the equal issue constantly. Machines and computers are designed to do repetitive duties.

The biggest supply of stress is other human beings. Maintaining suitable members of the family with human beings at work allows fantastically. Office parties, organization lunches and glad hours all assist to loosen up in each different's organization. A large a part of paintings stress is demanding approximately losing our jobs. This is natural. Office politics exchange, reorganizations show up, human beings get fired. I discover the handiest manner to loosen up on this surroundings is realize that I will usually get a task in a month or , if I lose this process. This helps me to cognizance on the paintings at hand and no longer worry approximately losing my task.

Office politics is never ending. I realized that the best time this ends is after I go away this process. And then I surprise why it mattered so much. I in my opinion keep away from it. This helps it less complicated for me to get my process executed.

I additionally discover that taking my lunch hour faraway from my workplace and faraway from my coworkers helps. I usually enjoy having lunch with other buddies, former coworkers. This enables to break out from office politics.

I also make it a factor no longer to take paintings home. If you should paintings remotely, discover some other location far from home to paintings. Coffee shops, internet cafes or network paintings areas are great. Working and gambling within the identical place isn't proper for the spirit. And it prevents me from enjoyable. Always take into account that 1/2 the a laugh of running is the relationships that I increase with people I paintings with. I commonly attempt to broaden long relationships with coworkers.

A forty hour work week is more than all of us can accomplish. The after hours must be spent enhancing relationships with people, time with family, pastimes and so forth. These add intensity to someone and make existence greater fun.

Clutter in workspace represents clutter within the head. So it is a good concept to periodically go through all the shelves and drawers and smooth out muddle. It is likewise a terrific idea to clear out unwanted file folders to your laptop

Driving is unavoidable in contemporary existence. I try to limit the amount of driving I do. If I'm on a job this is over 10 miles from domestic, I try to use public shipping or strive a far flung working association. Anything to lessen riding. I personally on-line delivery of as many stuff as feasible. That consists of groceries and almost the whole lot else. If I have to force lengthy distances, I preserve to a most of four hours using a day. I try to take a ten minute destroy each hour or so. This enables to loosen up the eyes.

In present day life-style is so smooth amassing matters and cluttering up my condominium. I select donating and freely giving as a whole lot as viable. This is less difficult than organizing or getting more objects to assist organizing. These are more things in my residence and upload to the litter. Fewer things make contributions to a feeling of area in my apartment. Interestingly simplifying my condominium facilitates to resolve my mind. I believe that items we keep are reflective of the chaos in our minds.

I also find that decluttering also constantly more space to extra around, and strive new thoughts. Interestingly this additionally helps to clear area in my thoughts and emerge as extra innovative. According to the

 Vastu Shastra, one's domestic and paintings location is one's temple. It is a spiritual region for us to live, breather and revel in our time in the world.

After work, the most important supply of strain is troubles with cutting-edge and former pals, circle of relatives, and full-size others. Whatever the reasons, enhancing relationships or simply absolutely casting off them from my existence, helps me to reduce the noise and chatter in my head. And this allows me to chill out appreciably.

Many of us could say that our cause for residing is to be glad. And to me, meaning absence of noises in my head. Most of these noises are self inflicted.

If a person made $40,000 a yr, and his pals and neighbors half of that, he might don't forget himself to be glad. If however his pals made greater than that, he could remember himself unhappy. One smart, guy as soon as stated, that a rich man is a person who makes $a hundred more than his spouse's sister's husband! We can drastically alternate our happiness via deciding who we examine ourself too. Am I better off, via comparing myself to my friend who made one million on internet shares or do I examine myself to a friend who earns minimum salary.

Many in modern-day society suppose that they might be happy by amassing big amount of wealth or being bodily healthy or by using having the good buddies. However, inspite of these, one can not be happy with out the right mindset. All people recognise of a person who has all of it, however is never glad. As the Dalai Lama says, "The real antidote to greed is contentment"/ Happiness facilitates to relax and with a extra comfortable thoughts, vision improves.

How will we obtain contentment? We need to be happy with what we've got. Desire best what can be finished. Contentment additionally relates to how much we price our self. Low self confidence consequences in low contentment. High self esteem is a supply of happiness, while the entirety else is gone. Happiness that relates to physical pleasures is brief and causes pressure. True happiness comes from the thoughts, and now not from the outside.

Pleasure and happiness are two various things. Pleasure follows happiness, instead of the other way round.

We do require basic needs to be satisfied. Food, apparel and shelter are a must. Anything extra than so as to now not deliver us happiness. To be glad, one wishes to get rid of all bad thoughts and feelings. This needs to be done one notion or emotion at a time. Quoting the Dalai Lama, the first step to being happy is getting to know.

A massive a part of strain is due to undesirable activities. A massive part of those occasions can be removed, through removing the reason. It takes time, however can be finished.

One of the relevant concepts of japanese philosophy is the precept of causality. Essentially it manner, what goes round, comes round. Or positioned in a different way, be nice to human beings in your way up, so they'll be quality to you for your way down. If you give happiness and pleasure, they come lower back. Hatred jealousy and anger are harmful. Compassion, warm temperature, and a type coronary heart, make one healthy and calm. One of the keys to attain calmness and lowering stress is adopting the proper mental mind-set.

This is much like training for a game. It includes more than simply popping nutrients.

It involves method, and exercise. And right mental conditioning.

Through repeated exercise of maintaining calmness, all disturbances arise at the floor, and by no means truely affect us. This enables to keep a calmness of thoughts. Interestingly as our minds get calmer, feelings of love and compassion stand up certainly. Human nature is largely compassionate and mild. All resources of aggression arise inside the mind and misuse of human intelligence.

Human beings are born satisfied. All toddlers bring to the joy to the sector and themselves. As we become old, human intelligence overpowers this and loss of pleasure. Purpose of existence is happiness.

The tendency to paintings collectively for the common precise is deeply ingrained in us. This is the essential premise of modern organizations and all business offers.

It is said that New York is the loneliest region in America. Imagine one in every of the largest metros in the world is so lonely. This is because of the inability to consciousness our consciousness outward and spot the first-class in each person. This on my own will cure all loneliness. People vibe socially, and this bonding contributes to our feeling of well being and happiness. Most of assume different people to take the initiative. A exchange of mindset is all it takes to treatment this.

In western tradition, dependency is seemed down upon. Independence is quite valued. So many overlook that the meals we eat comes the paintings of others. Clothing, housing and everything we use, comes from the paintings of others. This interconnectedness makes us alive and the dominant species on the planet.

Many folks are seeking out that one special individual, who would make us whole and complete. This is far an excessive amount of to assume from all and sundry. This form of standpoint is highly proscribing, and cuts us off from a wide style of intimate relationships. Instead compassion and reference to all people makes us whole and complete. Intimate attachments are the axle around which our lives revolve.

The definitions of intimacy vary throughout subculture and throughout time. However what has now not modified is the actual intimacy. Human beings nonetheless engage and connect the same manner over the millennia. This explains why the lessons of religious publications and the Kama Sutra are nonetheless legitimate. We need to boom our definition of intimacy to include each person, in place of focusing on the unique someone.

One way to connect is to position ourselves within the different man or woman's position. Imagine the individual listening to us and reacting to us. This approach might help to growth warmth and compassion to others.

Even if I have no not unusual floor with a stranger, it's clean to don't forget that everybody need to paintings, go to highschool, pay taxes and have all the matters that make us human.

All lengthy relationships are constructed on mutual consider and information. Some relationships are primarily based on certain commonalities. Friends at paintings, enterprise companions or sexual gratifications. These give up while the underlying basis is removed. Happiness is in part derived from the character and intensity of relationships, rather than acquiring fabric goods. Romance is brilliant, but it ought to no longer be the only source of happiness. When in love, one starts offevolved deceiving oneself and then starts deceiving others.

Genuine compassion for others implies forgiveness and expertise. This way non-aggression and non-controlling. Love implies freedom. Genuine love and authentic compassion is all pervading, deep and profound. And an extreme source of happiness. Genuine compassion involves an expertise of struggling.

The Dalai Lama says that we have to accept struggling part of existence, and tackle the problems that arise. Instead of ignoring it, it's far higher to confront. This is similar to understanding the skills of the enemy during battle and tackling troubles head on. Preparing oneself in advance for calamities makes one better organized to deal with it. Understanding that blurry vision happens due to strain within the thoughts and body, you'll reduce or keep away from unnecessary stresses.

Feelings of grief and anxiety are herbal. Problems arise while left unchecked. When extended depression consequences. In western societies grief, suffering and physical disabilities have been decreased or placed out of sight, to be cared for by health experts. Many anticipate that contamination and physical problems are not everyday. However in many poorer international locations, human beings are cared for by way of their circle of relatives and network. Suffering is taken into consideration to be a everyday human kingdom, to be understood and tackled. This allows to create peace of mind.

A large part of suffering is self created. In the "art of happiness", Howard Cutler offers this example of a man who nonetheless has sturdy emotions because of his spouse's infidelity. This endured even after being divorced for 17 years. We can add to our pain through being greater sensitive and overreacting to minor things. And taking matters in my view for minor infractions. And not reacting to important activities. Minor events have to bypass over us, like a leaf bending in the wind. Unhappiness is the result of being imprisoned in our own thoughts.

Problems usually come. If we cope with the trouble immediately then the trouble turns into a task. However if we upload the emotional component of "unfairness" suffering outcomes.

In Eastern philosophies there may be the law of Karma. What is going round comes around. However this doesn't avert action taken to make sure a end result. Too many hold out waiting for god or the authorities to shop them.

Our ordinary tendency is accountable others and outside factors. We also try to area the blame on a unmarried motive, instead of a large number of reasons, that's normally what takes place. Everything occurs due to the fact everything inside the universe has willed it to occur.

All of us are imperfect. All people have devoted mistakes. The regrets ought to not degenerate into excessive guilty. Holding directly to the past, reasons by no means finishing self punishment. Guilt arises while we are convinced that we have made an irreparable damage. Everything in lifestyles changes. Nothing is everlasting. However many of us face up to alternate in place of going with the glide. If we outline our self-picture via past accomplishments or what we used to appear to be, we develop unhappier as we become old. The more we hold on, greater hard existence turns into.

Relationships trade too. Levels of intimacy and passion differ. This is a ordinary sample of increase and improvement. This does now not mean developing apart. It is part of the cycle of clearing up old particles to start a new cycle of closeness.

Hardship by myself does no longer confer knowledge. Change of angle and introspection is what makes the distinction. Everything is relative. For one concept to exist the contrary has to exist. Heaven can not exist with out hell. Wealth can not exist with out poverty. Happiness can't exist with out disappointment. Looking at each laid low with the opposite perspectives allows to lessen the magnitude and can even rework the tragedy to a boon. This enables to lessen anger at a person while on can see different fantastic traits. Everything in live is in sun shades of gray. Everything and all of us has a few hell and heaven in them.

I lived through the first gulf struggle. I relocated to India and changed into a foreigner. At that point that turned into a tragedy. Twenty years later I learnt to get a greater international outlook. I learnt to be a neighborhood everywhere. And most importantly the attachment to fabric objects vanished. I became loose.

It is usually considered patriotic to hate one's enemy. This is said to improve national spirit. This is very dangerous and typically ends in conflict and enrichment of a select few. Who is an enemy and who's a pal is a matter of angle. If you don't believe me have a look at the international locations who're American allies. A huge wide variety of them were enemies inside the remaining hundred years.

Developing compassion for enemies is one of the keys to develop compassions for all. That changes an enemy to a non-enemy and maybe someday a pal. According to the Dalai Lama, that is intently interwoven with persistence and tolerance. There not any fortitude just like endurance simply as there's no discomfort worse than hatred. An enemy is necessary to examine endurance.

One of the keys to reducing strain is have a bendy questioning thoughts. The mind thinks in grooves. Thinking inside the identical sample reasons friction and pressure. Shifting perspectives and thinking out of the field enables clear up troubles and calms the thoughts.

However that stated, one among the most important stress relievers is to be congruent. Congruency implies a fixed of fixed fundamental beliefs around which one's lifestyles revolves. This makes it simpler to make decisions and less difficult for others to hook up with me.

Another key detail to dwelling a glad existence is stability. Buddha defines this as taking the middle direction. Living lifestyles in the facet can be a laugh, but can cause other imbalances. Exercise moderately is right, however beyond a factor results in serious accidents. Too a good deal or too little daylight can kill a plant.

It's smooth to get over excited by means of one's accomplishments and discouraged with the aid of suffering. It's appropriate to take into account difficulties in times of abundance and bear in mind the accomplishments in instances of famine. This restores balance. One of the motives for living the extremes is narrow mindedness. Pushing the boundaries may be emotionally exhilarating but can be dangerous to others or maybe me.

Victor Frankl stated that guy's purpose in life is to locate which means. A character can shoulder distress if he can locate which means in it.

There is a difference among bodily ache and intellectual pain. Mental pain is self inflicted by way of the mind. That can be cured through a exchange of perspective. Physical ache is to shield us from extra accidents. Leprosy patients don't sense pain. It is stated that a affected person ought to sleep peacefully even as someone is making an attempt to chop his limbs off!

Chapter 7: Money

Money is traumatic. Earning it, managing it, spending it. And the guidelines keep changing. The industrial revolution furnished a wealth of products at inexpensive fees. Large groups have been fashioned to produce and distribute those goods. More selections intended more pressure seeking to decide.

Universities have been created to teach professionals for these big organizations. For the primary time in history, human beings were pushed into a nine to 5 till 65 recurring. More stress. Then pension finances beginning disappearing, following via disappearance of process balance. Now its task hopping and pension plans. More pressure.

Once upon a time, earning a residing meant that living was the give up intention. And then earning became the give up goal. Soon forty hours had been now not sufficient. Add on the time to go back and forth, get dressed, attend paintings seminars, organisation socials, money control, our lives got ate up by means of paintings. More strain.

It's smooth to forget about how much we spend simply to live hired. We paintings harder and extra simply to hold the process. When I do my budget for the yr, I see that nearly 70% of my expenditure includes, rent, vehicle and decompression from paintings. If I didn't have a process, I could pay some distance less for rent, now not very own a car, and not invest in after paintings decompression sports, I could have to paintings much less tough and be less pressured.

The manner to deal with cash is to get a financial education. This involves learning to the way to make greater, how to control it and spend it wisely. This includes spending much less, saving extra, and making an investment wisely.

Consider the common employee. Up at 7 am, dress up professionally, fight rush hour traffic, be agreeable the entire day, wait to hurry out and try to decompress. This is incomes for demise.

Unfortunately that is the fact of existence. The strain may be notably decreased, however better courting management at work, and higher monetary management. By slicing down fees and making an investment wisely, passive profits grows. There is a crossover factor while the passive profits exceeds costs. This is a time for birthday celebration.

Sadly paintings becomes our identification rather a way. Many can in no way permit cross. Work will become our primary allegiance, our number one source of love and self expression. Along with racism and sexism, we now have jobism. Discrimination based totally on jobs. I had a communication with my dad and mom the opposite day: "All my friends' youngsters at the moment are presidents and VP. You're just a worker". "But ma, I make extra money that the ones presidents". "Arun, they have reputation, you don't!" Does this sound acquainted?

Even even though the common man or woman works more, and earns greater, he has much less money within the financial institution. There are times within the recent beyond, the countrywide savings fee has gone bad. Due to high mortgages, credit card debt, college bills and vehicle bills, we can not have the funds for to lose a task. We make a loss of life at paintings, to stay it up on the weekend.

Author Jeff Yaeger of "Cheapskate's manual to riches", recommends skipping the cash step totally. Many work harder to earn extra cash to visit a fitness center. However with lesser work, and greater manual labor at home, it's miles feasible to pass the extra hours. And get exercising transferring the garden or doing yoga at home.

We think we work to pay the bills. Instead we spend on stuff don't need. And extra paintings to get more money to get extra stuff. We suppose we need more money to be glad. Numerous research have shown that when a certain threshold, extra cash doesn't purchase happiness. This compares with studies executed on lottery winners. Very few felt any extra happiness.

It's time to say sufficient. I went via a binge buying segment. At the cease I had a filled up condominium sufficient for 2 households. I stopped spending. Interestingly, I felt heavier and slower. All these things simply filled by means of condominium and my mind. I commenced sorting through and downsizing. Almost 70% went out. I abruptly felt lighter and extra energetic than I had in years.

When the commercial age commenced, employees demanded and got shorter work weeks. The powers that be, have been alarmed that people have been enjoying their amusement, and no longer inclined to shop for. The customer changed into created. New markets were created from inside. The time period "fashionable of dwelling" turned into coined. Buying an increasing number of became equated with an elevated preferred of dwelling. The rat fee began. "Right to Buy" became the brand new fundamental right.

Buying have become a patriotic duty, to preserve the economic system going. Consumers no longer buying became sufficient to reason a depression. Disposable profits needed to be disposed. Advertisements completely surround. How are we able to no longer purchase?

To keep away from the cash lure, it's far vital to make small steps. A monetary training is a must. It is a sad reflection that the basics are in no way taught at college or university. Instead talking about cash is taboo. We feel unloved, we buy something. When we display our love, we buy some thing. We are bored, we purchase something. After all this, we wishfully don't forget the satisfied student days! The manner to avoid the cash trap is to say enough.

And what does this more buying convey? More litter.

Clutter is some thing that is excess for you. Anything that takes up space but doesn't serve you. Letting go off muddle is to open area interior of you. Decluttering improves alertness creativity and freedom.

A little recognised economist Paretto, created called the 80-20 rule. It essentially manner that 80% of consequences happen because of 20% of the inputs. So 80% of the stuff used is due to 20% of the stuff. 80% of our money comes from 20% of the results. Eighty% of manufacturing defects occur because of 20% of the problems. So focusing at the 20% improves productiveness and decreases muddle.

What causes clutter? It happens while we recognize that greater is better. It has been variously recommended that this a part of advertising and marketing campaigns and authorities supported advertising and marketing.

Many reasons have been recommended for the stop of the exquisite melancholy. One of the broadly attributed reasons is due to the multiplied spending of the US military at some stage in the Second World War. Since the give up of the conflict implied stop of colonies, domestic thrift became discouraged and those have been encouraged to spend more and more. A term "wellknown of residing" turned into coined. This basically supposed that greater is higher, despite the fact that it reasons muddle. Everyone is recommended to borrow more and spend greater.

I heard this thrilling story from a pal. His grandpa sold a piece of land within the Midwest for cash, and constructed the house himself. His son took a mortgage and paid it off in 5 years. His Dad didn't approve the hobby payments. My buddy paid off his house in 10 years. Again dad and grandpa didn't approve. Now his son has taken a forty 12 months loan! This is the sign of times. More debt for getting greater junk.

As your attention of clutter deepens, you'll begin cleaning out your complete life. I rearranged my price range, consolidated 4 401K plans into one, downsized 80%, deleted 80% of the emails cope with and phone numbers and also wiped clean the clutter on my paintings desk. Less stress.

As a primary step, it's miles useful to get a list of lifetime profits. This must include all earnings ever. Next it's far useful to take an stock of all belongings. Assents include something that generates earnings or may be bought. This calls for complete honesty. It's unexpected I have earned and what sort of I actually have earned with the aid of promoting stuff online.

We're no longer incomes a dwelling. We're earning a demise. We work hard to store for retirement, so we can spend it. More pressure.

There are extraordinary viewpoints of cash. First is the road level view. This is the every day transactions. Then we've got the penthouse view. This is in which we take a view of our complete financial records. Then there may be the distance deliver view, wherein we take a look at the life power we trade our money for.

Money is some thing we trade our life power for. If we make $20 consistent with hour, we have traded 1 hour of our lifestyles for $20. So if we purchase some thing for $20, we've traded in a single hour of our lifestyles for that object. Just deliberating that, made me trade my perspective on money and paintings. Knowing this, what might you like to do with your existence electricity?

Financial independence normally way having greater wealth than my neighbors. In reality monetary independence is the revel in of getting sufficient. This is a figure that is achievable. This takes place while we study our budget from the distance ship view.

A 2nd step would be to maintain tune of all spending. I pay all my payments via credit score playing cards. I then use on line equipment to help me song my fees. This manner I can recognize all my monthly fees. It sudden in which I spend and on what.

It's easy to forget how a great deal cash we spend simply to have a process. I become startled to comprehend that I may want to reduce my expenditure through almost sixty percentage if I didn't have a task. The greater spending consists of living in an expensive place in the direction of work, go back and forth prices, ingesting out fees, clothing charges and decompression fees. The ultimate is the cash I spent to loosen up after paintings. This may include gyms, holidays or shopping.

Budgets don't paintings. Just like diets. I tried both, by no means succeeded. I determined that as I saved track of prices and looked at them frequently, I observed that I didn't want to finances. I robotically adjusted my spending. I additionally remind myself that I'm spending my existence electricity.

The way to hold eating and weight below control is to devour when hungry. And get normal workout. The quality manner to keep spending beneath manipulate is to spend simplest when required. And no longer take a look at commercials, or cling out on the mall.

Ask yourself. What do you need the money for? Is it time to write down the tremendous American novel? To become an artist? To journey the world? Or to mention simply have more than a few to reveal off? This tells you where the achievement curve truely is. Again ask your self, in case you received satisfaction and price in share to life power spent. Are you doing this due to the fact a person says so? Are you getting sufficient fulfillments from all of your prices and work? Looking at my prices I turned into under spending in art and music. And overspending in gadgets I in no way used. I felt better balanced.

Life energy flows within the direction of where we spend. Under spending in achievement and overspending on gazingus pins brings fewer fulfillments and greater stress. It is vital to develop an internal measure of achievement, to kick useless spending. Less spending means extra money inside the financial institution and faster retirement.